Transitioning to the NCLEX-RN®: Pharmacology Study Guide

Marnie L. Kramer-Kile RN, PhD

Kramer-Kile, M.L. (2015). Transitioning to the NCLEX-RN®: Pharmacology Study Guide (1st ed.)Kimberley, BC: Kramer-Kile Nurse Education Consultants Ltd.Registration No. 1125810.

Study Guide Design by Perpetual Notion, Edmonton, AB.

About the Author

Dr. Marnie Kramer-Kile is a nursing faculty member at the College of the Rockies in Cranbrook, British Columbia, Canada. An experienced undergraduate nurse educator and national speaker on RN registration exam preparation, Marnie has expertise in creating practical study approaches using exam competency frameworks and test plans as a guide. She has extensive experience in preparing Canadian graduates to write the previous Canadian Registered Nurse Exam (CRNE) and the current NCLEX-RN®. Marnie's passion is helping repeat writers of high stakes registration exams by creating study resources to help students take a more targeted approach to exam preparation. Marnie can be reached directly at marnie@rnstudyguides.ca

Table of Contents

Table of Contents

Module 1

Understanding Drug-to-Drug Interactions

TABLE OF CONTENTS

TABLE OF CONTENTS

Tables and Figures

Introduction to the Transitioning to the NCLEX-RN®: Pharmacology Study Guide Module 1: Drug-to-Drug Interactions

The breadth and detail of the knowledge required of pharmacological concepts often overwhelms new graduates when they are beginning their exam preparation. The purpose of this pharmacology study guide is to help you work through the vast amount of pharmacological knowledge required for the NCLEX-RN® in a systematic and purposeful way. This guide organizes content using the current NCLEX-RN® Test Plan and provides specific strategies to address pharmacological areas of review which may challenge new graduates. **This is the first of twelve modules.** This is a working guide, so while key information will be presented and organized for review, it is up to you to do the detailed work of content review by answering the questions and exercises in each Module. You can expect to see drugs described by their generic names on the exam. Due to the differences in drug trade names between the United States of America, Canada and other nations you should study drugs according to their generic names and develop strategies for remembering them.

This module is part of a comprehensive pharmacology study guide focusing on specific areas which may challenge NCLEX-RN® candidates. This includes drug-to-drug interactions, specific adverse reactions due to drug therapy and the potential reactions associated with herbal therapy and conventional medications. The content will be focused on a systems approach and will direct you towards important information within each drug class.

Structure of the Guide

This guide begins with a review of the basics of pharmacological therapy: pharmacokinetics, pharmacodynamics, and an overview of the differing drug classes for each body system will be highlighted in order to provide a structure for review. Additional areas for review that are specialized or affect multiple systems will also be highlighted:

1. Review questions and selected exercises will be constructed for each drug class to help pull out key concepts such as adverse events/side effects, specific client teaching and drug to drug interactions.
2. A summary chart of the drug classes in each system or theme will be provided for you to use alongside practice questions. As you move through practice questions, check off the specific medications you come across and if you require further review in each area. It is also helpful to make your own drug cards for specific medications. Keep the drug cards simple. Identify the drug class, the mechanism of action, two relevant (i.e., life threatening) or unique adverse effects that require monitoring and provide an outline for client teaching or specific nursing interventions for the medication.

Advice for Studying Pharmacological Content for the NCLEX-RN®

Always start with areas you are NOT familiar with. For example, if you spent the majority of your time as a final practicum student on a cardiology unit do not start in the Vascular and Cardiac Medications Module. It is common for students/graduates to move to areas of comfort when they are studying because it decreases their anxiety. However, your efforts should be targeted on what you don't know. Each Module in this guide has a summary table of drugs for each system. Highlight first the drug classes that you are not familiar with and make it your priority to work through them. Do not spend time making drug cards for medications you already know. For example, most students are confident with furosemide administration and can critically think through concepts associated with the drug. Only make drug cards for medications that are new to you. The review questions in this guide will direct you towards more detailed information of the medications that you are familiar with and focus on potential areas where exam questions may be asked.

This guide is set up using a **systems approach** for the following reasons: 1) most pharmacology textbooks use this approach to structure content so it will be easier to find the information you need to answer the review questions; 2) using a systems approach allows you to find commonalties in the side effects of drugs influencing a specific system, so you will see patterns arising as you work through this guide; and 3) a systems approach allows for the creation of overall drug summary tables, which will be included in each module of the guide and will provide you with a general sense of the medications you need to cover.

The following resources will aid you in answering questions posed in this guide. This includes:

1. **A pharmacology textbook.** This resource will contain more detailed information pertaining to drug classes and outline general nursing considerations for therapy. I have referenced a pharmacology textbook throughout the writing of this guide.
2. **A drug guide**. These are the guides commonly used for your clinical practice. These resources contain alphabetized drug information. Most importantly, they outline specific pharmacokinetic and pharmacodynamics properties of drugs. You will find information related to drug excretion, protein binding, and therapeutic index in these guides.
3. **An online drug repository** for more detailed information that may not be found in the two resources above. Sometimes it is difficult to find therapeutic index and protein binding for a drug. I have found the following website helpful for this: http://www.drugbank.ca/drugs

Module 1: Understanding Drug-to-Drug Interactions

This first module provides strategies for approaching content related to drug-to-drug interactions in the context of the NCLEX-RN® exam. Candidates often struggle with this content on the exam, however, there are specific strategies to help work through these types of exam questions. Rather than spending hours attempting to *memorize* specific drug-to-drug interactions candidates can learn to *think critically* through this content and pull out important pieces of information required to answer exam questions successfully. In order to do so, it is imperative that you understand the concepts of pharmacokinetics and pharmacodynamics and the role these concepts play in drug interactions. Before you begin studying in this section, ensure that you review and understand the concepts outlined in the review questions below. You will find the answers to these questions in your pharmacology textbook utilized in your nursing program.

REVIEW QUESTIONS

Pharmacokinetics and Pharmacodynamics

1. Define the term “pharmacokinetics”. Describe the phases of absorption, distribution, biotransformation and excretion in relation to drug therapy.
2. What factors influence drug absorption? What is the “first pass” effect?
3. What is the difference between drugs that are lipid or water soluble?
4. How does ionization affect drug absorption? Are drugs better absorbed when they are ionized or non-ionized?
5. Define the term “bioavailability”.
6. How does pH influence drug absorption? Provide an example.
7. Why is it important to know if a drug is bound to protein? What does it mean when a drug is 99.5% protein bound? How does this influence drug dosing?
8. What is the Hepatic Microsomal Enzyme System (P450 system)? How does it influence the biotransformation of medications? (Important: knowledge of this system is essential in understanding drug-to-drug interactions)
9. Identify potential sites of drug excretion in the body.
10. Define the term “pharmacodynamics”. In the context of drug-receptor interactions define what agonist, antagonist and agonist-antagonist drugs are.
11. What are drug-enzyme interactions? What are some other examples of non-specific drug reactions in the body?
12. What is the difference between potency and efficacy of medications?
13. What is a therapeutic index? Why is this important for drug therapy? Are drugs more dangerous if they have a low or high therapeutic index?
14. What is *half-life* in the context of drug therapy? Why is it important to know a drug's half-life?

STUDYING CONTENT FOR DRUG-TO-DRUG INTERACTIONS

When two drugs interact there are three possible outcomes (Rosenjack Burchum & Rosenthal, 2016, p.55)

1. One drug may **intensify** the effects of the other (increased therapeutic effects OR increased adverse effects)
2. One drug may **reduce** the effects of the other (reduced therapeutic effects OR reduced adverse effects)
3. The combination may produce a **new response** not seen with either drug alone

Remember when approaching NCLEX-RN® exam questions regarding drug-to-drug interactions that there are <u>four possible ways that drugs can interact with each other</u>:

1. **Direct chemical or physical interaction**—most commonly seen in IV solutions, precipitate may form. To avoid this, never combine two or more drugs in the same IV bag unless it has been established that a direct interaction will NOT occur.
2. **Pharmacokinetic interactions**—through mechanisms of altered drug absorption, altered drug distribution, altered metabolism, altered renal excretion or interactions that involve p-glycoprotein.
3. **Pharmacodynamic interactions**—interactions at the same receptor or interactions resulting from actions at separate sites.
4. **Combined Toxicity**—both drugs have toxic effects on the same organ.

The next two figures (Figures 1.1, 1.2) review the basics of drug administration and identify pharmacological concepts. Review the difference between pharmacokinetics and pharmacodynamics along with the associated terminology in each section. These concepts will help you to learn to pick out the most dangerous drugs in NCLEX-RN® questions and help you to identify potential interactions even if you only have knowledge of one of the drugs identified in the question.

Figure 1.1: Approaching Pharmacological Therapy Map

The goal of care during states of illness is to restore homeostasis and help the body to adapt—cells are the building blocks and the most important part of our bodies. Always think: "What is happening at a cellular level?"

What is a drug?

↓

Drugs can help or harm the body

↓

Nurses must gain knowledge about drug administration

↓

Nurses must know about the: patient (age, present condition, co-morbidities, attitude towards taking medications, ability to take or swallow medications, level of consciousness);pathology affecting the patient; why the medication is being ordered; agency policies surrounding medication administration; legal responsibilities (includes scope of practice); and ethical issues surrounding the drug.

↓

A physician or nurse practitioner (Health Care Provider) order is required for drug administration. These may be single, stat, prn, standing or continuing orders. The order must have the drug name, dose, route, time and frequency of medication. For example: diphenhydramine 25mg, po, q6h, prn.

↓

Nurses must be able to protect patients from unsafe orders by knowing the 1) Indication, 2) Dosage, 3) Side Effects, 4) Adverse Effects and 5) Nursing Implications for each drug.

↓

Always assess the patient, order and hospital policy prior to giving a drug

↓

Identify existing or anticipated problems with drug administration

↓

Set goals for care

↓

Administer the drug, keeping in mind: 10 rights of medication administration, 3 checks, and always document immediately

↓

Evaluate the drug and its effectiveness

Figure 1.2 Pharmacokinetics and Pharmacodynamics

Pharmaceutical Phase:

Drug must be dissolved before it can be absorbed.
What is the effect on varying volumes of water ingested on oral drug absorption?
How does drug preparation affect absorption?

Pharmacokinetics (Movement of Drug)

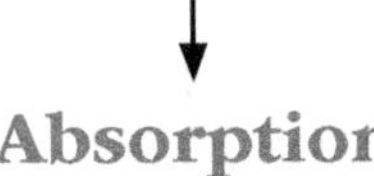

Absorption

(Drug moves from site of administration to the blood)
All drugs must cross the plasma membrane through:
-active transport (also called specialized transport)
- passive transport (also called simple diffusion)
- pinocytosis

Drug molecules may be: Ionized (requires active transport, water soluble) or non-ionized (simple diffusion and lipid soluble)
Factors affecting the absorption of drugs: circulation to site of administration, absorbing membranes, drug composition, solubility of drug, pH, ionic charge of drug molecule.
What is meant by the term bioavailability?
What can the nurse do to enhance drug absorption?

Distribution

(Drug moves from blood to site of action)
Distribution is affected by blood supply, drug's affinity to the receptor, ionization of drug, plasma protein binding.
What is meant by plasma protein binding?

Biotransformation

(Drug changed from one form to another)
Helps to facilitate excretion of the drugs
What is the first pass effect?
What is the role of the Hepatic Microsomal Enzyme System?
Which factors affect biotransformation?

Excretion

(Drug is removed from the body)
What are the sites of excretion in the body? What factors influence renal drug excretion?
What does the kidney NOT filter out of the body? How does the pH of the filtrate in the kidney influence drug excretion?
What are some foods that affect urine pH?

Pharmacodynamics

(Drug Action – how the drug changes the body)

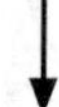

Drugs interact with particular molecules, modify existing function, and produce both desired and, at times, undesired effects

All Drugs affect cells by one of the following mechanisms:

1. **Drug-Receptor Interaction** (drug combines with receptor on or in a cell)
Drugs can bind to receptors and act as: **agonists** (drug binds to receptor to produce and action), **antagonists**(binds to a specific receptor and prevents other drugs/substances from producing an action) or as a **competitive antagonist** (two drugs compete for the same receptors, decreasing one another's action).
- Which types of drugs then will have fewer side effects?

2. **Drug Enzyme Interaction** (drug combines with enzymes in the cell)
This usually results in the drug changing pharmacokinetic factors (i.e., absorption, distribution, biotransformation or excretion)

3. **Non-Specific Drug Action**
Drugs may be used to replace deficient nutrients, alter the function of the cell or cause chemical reactions.

- What is the difference between potency and efficacy?
- What is meant by the term "steady state" when talking about drug action?
- All drug therapy must be monitored; this is done by monitoring the level of the drug in the plasma.
- Describe the difference between the therapeutic range and the therapeutic index of a drug.
- How does half-life influence drug dosing? How is the dosing of the drug adjusted for patients with hepatic or renal failure?

Pharmacogenetics (Role of heredity in drug response)

Understanding how Drug-to-Drug Interactions Occur

The principle of ionization is important in understanding how drugs can potentially interact with each other. Non-ionized drugs pass easily through the cell membrane, while ionized drugs require active transport. If one drug (A) has the potential to decrease the ionization of another drug (B), Drug B becomes easier for the cell membrane to absorb. This can become problematic if Drug B is designed to be absorbed in a certain part of the digestive system (in the case of an oral drug) or if the fixed dose is designed for a drug that is known to be ionized. Drug B can increase to high levels in the blood due to rapid absorption. An example would be with antacids that elevate gastric pH; in this case the more alkaline environment in the stomach influences the ionization of any other oral drugs given (Rosenjack Burchum et al, 2016, p.56). Other ways that absorption can be influenced in drug-to-drug interactions include (p.56):

1. Reduction of regional blood flow to the area of absorption.
2. Drugs that accelerate other drugs passage through the intestines (e.g., laxatives).
3. Drugs that decrease other drugs passage through the intestines (e.g., morphine).
4. Drugs that induce vomiting
5. Absorbent drugs that are given orally but pass through the GI tract, which have the potential to absorb and excrete other drugs (e.g., cholestyramine)

STEP 1:Do any of the Drugs Posed in the Exam Question have the Potential to Affect the Absorption of the other Drugs?

Complete the following exercise below to help you understand the influence of drugs on absorption.

Exercise 1: Drugs Influencing Absorption

Become familiar with specific drugs that may influence drug absorption so you can immediately recognize them when writing the NCLEX-RN®. Complete a list of medications that might:

Decrease blood flow to the GI tract	
Increase peristalsis	
Decrease peristalsis	
Induce Vomiting	

If none of the medications in the exam question influence drug absorption, then you will move to the next strategy.

STEP 2: Does the Drug Alter Distribution?

Two primary mechanisms influence the distribution of drugs: 1) protein binding and 2) extracellular pH.

Protein Binding

It is important to know if a drug is protein bound. There are various types of protein in the blood that drugs can bind to. For the sake of simplicity in explaining this concept, we will focus on albumin as the primary protein. When a drug is absorbed into the bloodstream, a certain percentage of the drug binds to albumin, while the rest is free in the blood. Drugs that are bound to protein cannot leave the vascular space and can't be excreted. The free drug in the plasma is what crosses into the cells and causes the drug's action. The rest of the drug stays bound to the protein. When pharmacological companies develop drugs they determine the minimum effective dose based on the amount of free drug in the plasma. It is important to remember that albumin only has a limited number of sites for the drug to bind to (Rosenjack Burchum et al, 2016, p.34). Therefore, if another drug has the potential to compete for protein binding, it has the potential to increase free levels of other drugs in the plasma and cause toxic effects. Typically, in a client with normal kidney and liver function, this higher level of free drug is metabolized and excreted when this happens (p.56). However, if a client has renal or hepatic impairments drugs can reach toxic levels. Also, some drugs are dangerous if another drug competes for protein binding (e.g., Warfarin). A drug is considered highly protein bound if it is more than 99%. You will find information regarding protein binding for specific medications in your drug guide. It is important to include this information on your drug cards (an example is provided later in this module).

Extracellular pH

We will look at the concept of extracellular pH from two perspectives. The first is in the GI tract. In the example provided in Step 1, it was shown that drugs that change gastric pH can influence the ionization of drugs and their absorption in the GI tract. Second, changes in pH can also be manipulated to promote excretion of drugs in the urine. Drugs that are lipid soluble (non-ionized) are passively reabsorbed in the renal tubules back into the blood stream. Therefore, water soluble (ionized drugs) remain in the renal tubules to be excreted. If you can manipulate the ionization of a drug with another drug you can influence whether it is excreted faster or taken up by the body. The treatment of drug overdoses provides an example of this. Rosenjack Burcham et al. (2016) use the example of ASA overdose. In this case the client is treated with an agent that increases urinary pH (sodium bicarbonate), since ASA is an acidic drug it becomes ionized in an alkaline environment and is thereby moved out of the body by the kidneys.

STEP 3: Does the Drug Alter the Metabolism of Other Drugs?

This is one of the most complex mechanisms of drug-to-drug interactions. The majority of drug metabolism occurs through the P450 (CYP) enzyme system of the liver. It is overwhelming to look at the full list of drugs that are substrates, inhibitors or inducers of this system. Rather than go into the system in full detail, for the purpose of NCLEX-RN® preparation I will provide some basic strategies for studying drugs that may be influenced by this system in the context of drug-to-drug interactions.

The first step is to **always study the signs of toxicity of a drug.** Start with drugs that will cause severe harm or death when they are toxic. These are drugs with low therapeutic indexes. This means that the drug is dosed at a level that can cause toxicity if it is taken off balance. For example, if the regular metabolism of this drug is inhibited by another drug it will reach toxic levels. **Exercise 2** below identifies drugs with a low therapeutic index. Start by becoming familiar with these drugs and their signs of toxicity. Chances are that these will be the most common drugs on the exam in questions involving drug-to-drug interactions.

The second step is to **know the mechanism of action of the drug(s) in the question and the intended effects**. If the drug-to-drug interaction causes metabolism of the drug to speed up then you will not see the drug's intended effects on the body. For example, if a woman is taking oral contraceptives and phenobarbital, the phenobarbital speeds up the metabolism of the oral contraceptives. Therefore, the oral contraceptive would be moved from the body at a higher rate. You may find that the woman is experiencing spotting or early menstruation if the drug levels dropped too quickly. She would be at risk of becoming pregnant because of this drug-to-drug interaction.

STEP 4: Does the Drug have the Potential to Alter Renal Excretion?

Recall the example provided in Step 2 with ASA and sodium bicarbonate in the context of extracellular pH. Drugs and food can also influence urinary pH. This is an important concept to think with when approaching exam questions. Remember:

- Alkaline urine → acid drug excreted
- Acid urine → alkaline drug excreted

Table 1.1 Foods that Acidify or Alkalinize Urine

Foods that Acidify Urine	Foods that AlkalinizeUrine	
• Cranberries • Cheese • Eggs • Lentils • Pastas • Grains • Plums (Prunes)	• Milk • Vegetables • Fruits	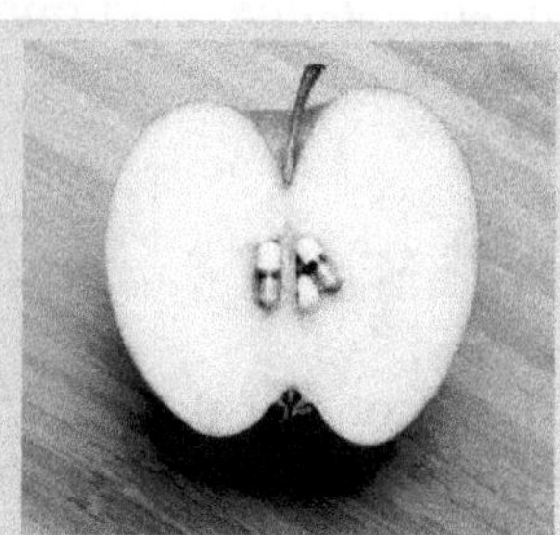

STEP 5: Identify Potential Pharmacodynamic Interactions

In this case, drugs may act on the same receptor site, interact at different sites or combine to produce toxic effects. Always think about the two drugs given in the exam question. What do you think is the worst thing that can happen if the drugs are combined? For example, if they are both anticoagulants, the client may be at an increased risk for bleeding; if they are both narcotic analgesics the client may experience respiratory depression. Also, it is important to prioritize one medication over the other. Which one is the most important to client care, and what happens if it becomes toxic or stops working? If drugs compete for the same receptor site, it will be evident that each drug has the potential to become toxic or be limited in its therapeutic action. If drugs interact at different receptor sites, rather than competing, they may have the potential to potentiate each other; again, study signs of toxicity of medications. Finally, think about potential toxicity to the kidneys and the liver when the drugs are combined. Are there any signs of renal or hepatic failure available as potential answers? It is helpful to pay careful attention to exam questions that focus on geriatric clients in acute care settings because this population, in particular, is at an increased risk of drug-drug interactions influenced by polypharmacy and altered renal or hepatic function (Lea et al., 2013).

Figures 1.3 and 1.4 provide summaries of the steps identified above. These figures may be helpful to use alongside your practice questions.

Figure 1.3: Approaching Exam Questions Pertaining to Drug-to-Drug Interactions

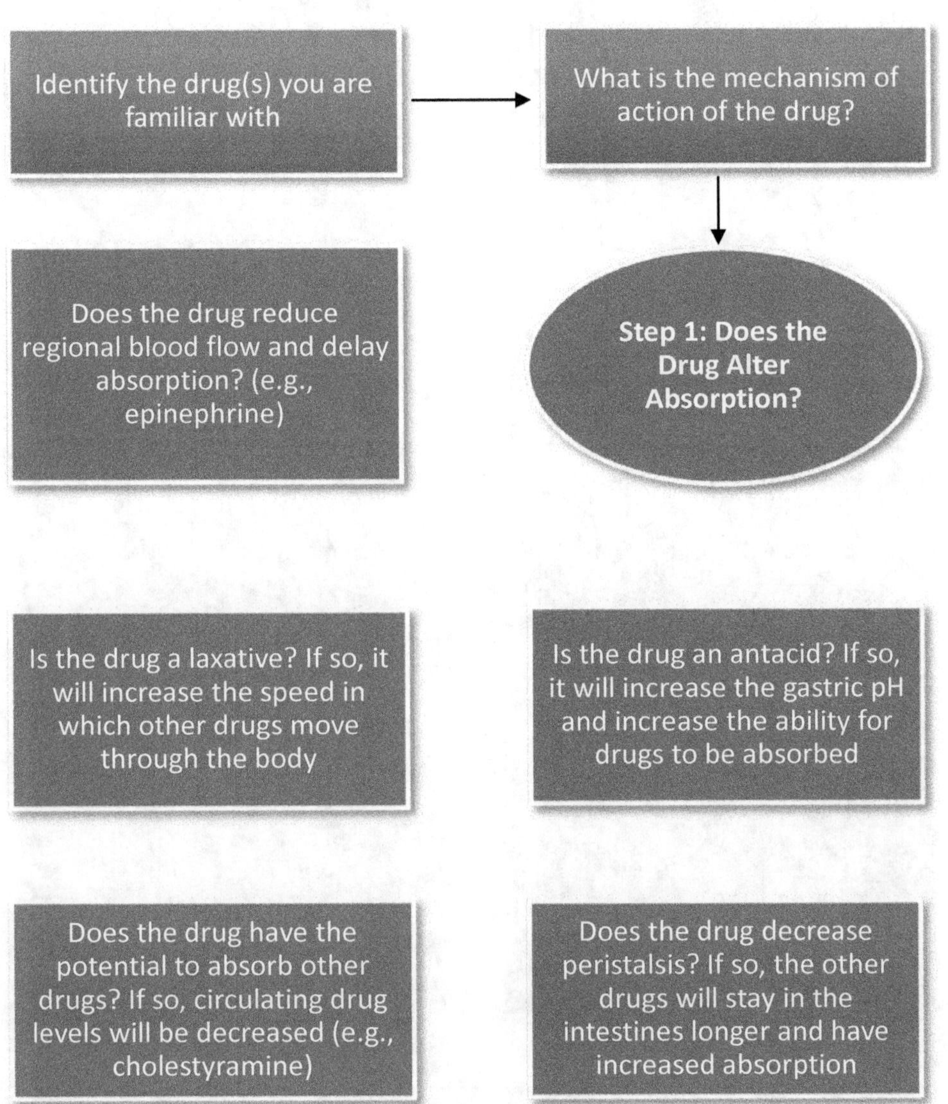

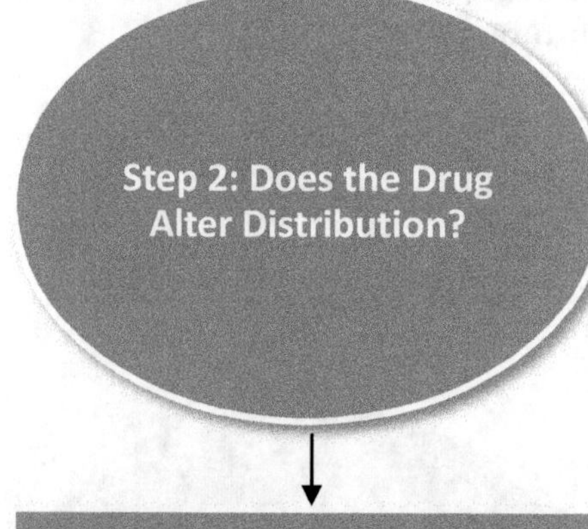
Step 2: Does the Drug Alter Distribution?

Is the drug highly protein bound? Meaning that it requires higher dosing because the majority of the drug binds to protein (e.g., albumin) and is excreted? When other drugs are given they can compete for protein binding. In this case you will see toxic effects of the drug.

↓

Does the drug alter extracellular pH? By increasing or decreasing extracellular pH, drugs will move in and out of cells.

Step 3: Does the Drug Alter Metabolism? Also, think about liver function (this is where the majority of interactions occur)

↓

Drugs will increase the metabolism of other drugs, therefore you will see DECREASED therapeutic effects in this case.

↓

Drugs will decrease the metabolism of other drugs, therefore you will see INCREASED therapeutic effects in this case.

Common Drug Classes Whose Metabolism is Altered by Other Drugs:

CNS drugs, antidysrhythmic drugs, beta blockers, opioids, antibacterials/antifungals, anticancer drugs, calcium channel blockers, drugs for HIV infection, sedative-hypnotics

See **Exercise 2** to help you with these concepts

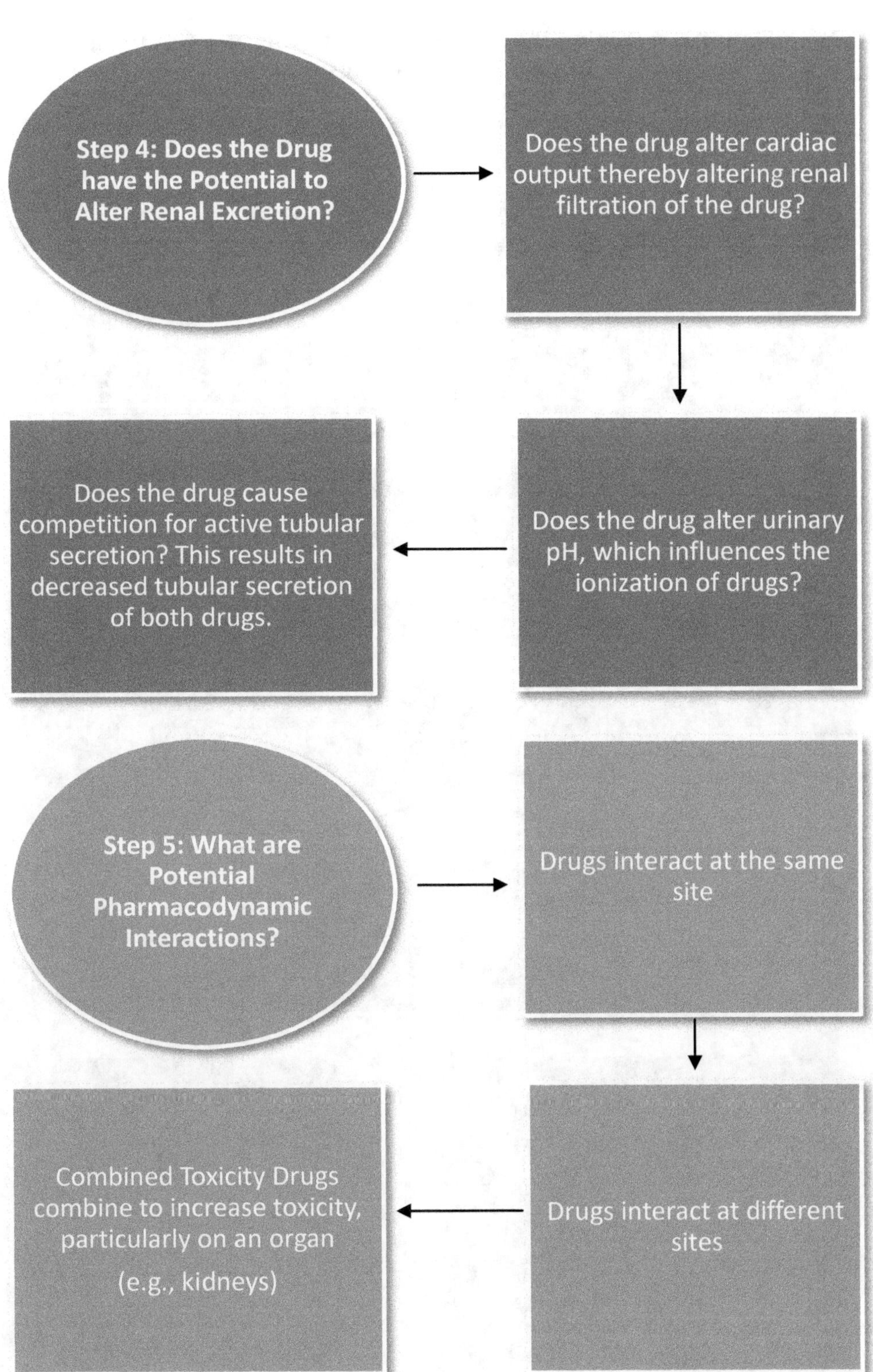
Step 4: Does the Drug have the Potential to Alter Renal Excretion?
Does the drug alter cardiac output thereby altering renal filtration of the drug?
Does the drug alter urinary pH, which influences the ionization of drugs?
Does the drug cause competition for active tubular secretion? This results in decreased tubular secretion of both drugs.
Step 5: What are Potential Pharmacodynamic Interactions?
Drugs interact at the same site
Drugs interact at different sites
Combined Toxicity Drugs combine to increase toxicity, particularly on an organ
(e.g., kidneys)

Figure 1.4: Putting it all Together: Answering Drug-to-Drug Interaction Exam Questions

Find the drugs you are familiar with in the question

Do any of the drugs in the question have a low therapeutic index? (increased risk for toxicity)

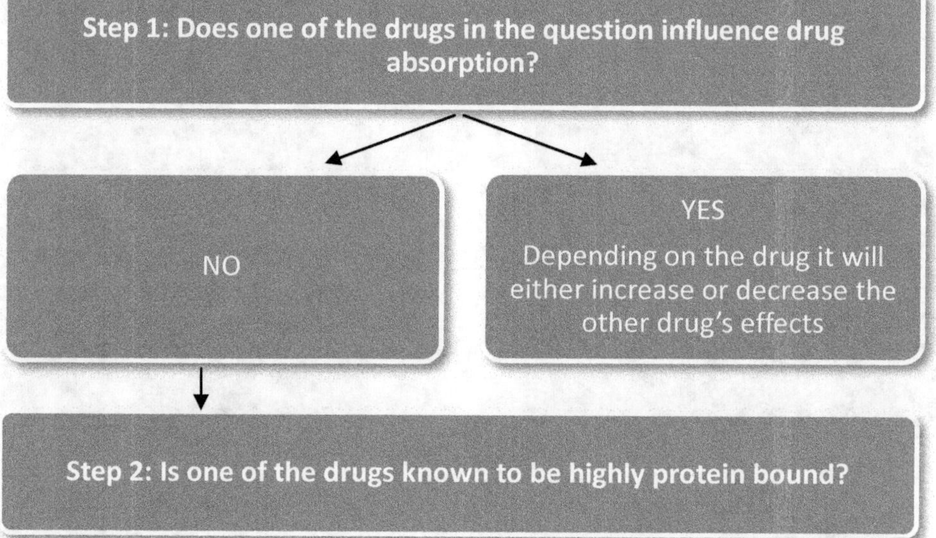
Step 1: Does one of the drugs in the question influence drug absorption?
NO
YES
Depending on the drug it will either increase or decrease the other drug's effects
Step 2: Is one of the drugs known to be highly protein bound?

NO

Step 3: Does the drug interact to alter the metabolism of other drugs?

YES

The drug interaction may cause increased plasma levels of one of the drugs. Look for signs of toxicity

YES

There is the potential for either decreased or Increased Effects—look at the information provided in the exam question to source out what is happening.

Consider Step 4: Renal function of client or the ability of the drug to influence ionization or urine pH

NO

Step 5: Do the drugs act on the same drug receptors? Or at different sites with the same effects?

Applying the Algorithm with a Practice Question:

The nurse is caring for a client who has been prescribed sucralfate. The nurse checks the client's medication history because the absorption of which of the following medication(s) can be affected if taken concurrently? **Select all that apply** (Silvestri, 2014, question 322).

1. Theophylline
2. Digoxin
3. Furosemide
4. Phenytoin
5. Warfarin Sodium

Sulcralfate coats the stomach and can delay absorption of other medications.

Which of the following medications are problematic if they do not follow the normal mechanism of absorption and remain available for longer? (Choose drugs with a narrow therapeutic index).

Theophylline, Digoxin, Phenytoin, Warfarin Sodium all have narrow therapeutic indexes, meaning they can rise to toxic levels quickly.

The nurse is caring for a client who has been prescribed sucralfate. The nurse checks the client's medication history because the **absorption** of which medication(s) can be affected if **taken concurrently**? Select all that apply (Silvestri, 2014, question 322).

1. **Theophylline**
2. **Digoxin**
3. Furosemide
4. **Phenytoin**
5. **Warfarin Sodium**

The remainder of this module focuses on exercises to help you gain familiarity with potential sources of drug-to-drug interactions. Complete the exercises below in order to better understand the concepts covered in the module and to become familiar with common medications that cause both food and drug-to-drug interactions.

Table 1.2 Explaining Drug-Food Interactions

Drug-Food Interactions

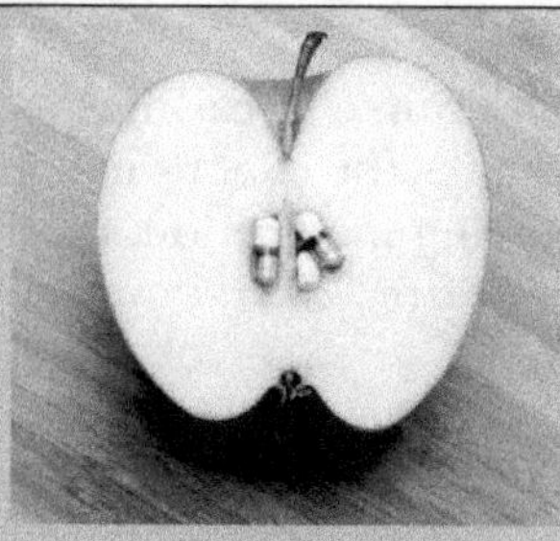

Drug to food interactions typically result in drug toxicity or therapeutic failure of the drug. In some cases, such as with foods containing tyramine that interact with MAOI's, the interaction can cause life-threatening physiological changes (e.g., hypertensive crisis). However, the primary mechanism of most drug-food interactions results in increased or decreased drug absorption. Grapefruit juice is a common food that inhibits the metabolism of drugs and raises their blood levels. Exercise 2 covers common drugs influenced by the consumption of grapefruit juice. Other significant examples include (p.59-60):

- Digoxin levels can be decreased by fibrous foods such as wheat bran, rolled oats, sunflower seeds.
- High calorie meals can increase the absorption of saquinavir (HIV medication) if the drug is not taken with food the drug is NOT well absorbed.
- Theophylline taken with caffeine can result in excessive CNS excitation.
- Spironolactone plus salt substitutes can result in dangerously high K+ levels.
- Aluminum-containing antacids plus citrus beverages can result in excessive absorption of aluminum.
- Foods containing Vitamin K can decrease the action of warfarin.

Drug-food reactions influencing drug absorption can be better managed by spacing out meals and drug administration as indicated. It is helpful to include on your drug cards if a drug should be taken on an empty or full stomach. When an order asks for a drug to be given on an empty stomach this means 1 hour before a meal or two hours after a meal (p.61).

Integrative Therapy Caution

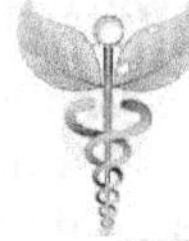

Herbal Medication: Echinacea

Changes the metabolism of many drugs that are affected by the CYP450 system leading to side effects or reduced effectiveness of medications (Richards, 2013).

Exercise 2: Drugs Levels Increased by Grapefruit Juice

Grapefruit juice when administered with medications always raises the drugs levels. Complete the following table to familiarize yourself with drugs that become toxic when administered with grapefruit juice.

Drug Name	Why is the drug given?	Assessment findings related to toxicity
Amlodipine		
Diltiazem		
Verapamil		
Simvastatin (includes all statin drugs)		
Amiodarone		
Carbamazepine		
Buspirone		
Midazolam		
Saquinavir		
Cyclosporine		
Sirolimus/tacrolimus		
SSRI medications (fluoxetine, sertraline)		
Dextromethorphan		
Sildenafil		

Understanding Therapeutic Index in the Context of Drug-to-Drug Interactions

Therapeutic response of drugs is directly related to their level in the plasma. (In most cases, it is impossible to measure the concentration of the drug at its target tissue). It is common for Health Care Providers to monitor drugs that have potentially harmful effects if their levels are too high. The **therapeutic range** of a drug is the drug concentration between the minimum effective range and the toxic concentration of the medication (Rosenjack Burchum et al., 2016, p.39). With some drugs, the therapeutic range is wide and there is more room to play with the dosage of the drug, while with others the range is quite narrow. The **therapeutic index** is used as a ratio of lethal dose to minimum effective dose (p.53). The **median lethal dose** is developed in pre-clinical trials is the dose of drug that will be lethal in 50% of a group of animals (Adams et al., 2008, p.58). It is divided by the median effective dose or ED 50 which is the dose required to produce a specific therapeutic response in 50% of a group of clients.

$$\text{Therapeutic ratio} = \frac{LD_{50}}{ED_{50}}$$

The closer the ratio is to 1 the greater the danger. The following table includes drugs with a known low therapeutic index (remember low is dangerous and a high therapeutic index is safer (Rosenjack Burchum et al., 2016, p.53).

Exercise 3: Identifying Drugs with Low Therapeutic Index

Complete the following table of drugs with a known low (dangerous) therapeutic index. Identify signs of toxicity of these medications. This will help you in picking out toxicity of these drugs in exam questions.

Drug Name	Mechanism of Action	Signs of Toxicity
Warfarin		
Levothyroxine		
Carbamazepine		
Lithium Carbonate		
Digoxin		
Phenytoin		
Theophylline		
Gentamicin		
Vancomycin		
Methotrexate		
Phenytoin		
Insulin		
Cyclosporine		

Changing your Study Strategies to Better Address Drug-to-Drug Interactions

Changing the focus of your drug cards can help you be better prepared for exam questions on drug-to-drug interactions. Figure 1.5 provides an example of this using Furosemide as a prototype drug. **Remember that it is beneficial to make your own cards rather than trying to memorize premade drug cards. Always make drug cards for drugs you are unfamiliar with first.** You do not need to spend time on drugs that you know well. It may help, however, to research concepts such as protein binding with common medications in order to help you address potential drug-to-drug interactions on the exam.

Figure 1.5 Example of Sample Drug Card for Studying (Rationale included)

Generic name:Furosemide **(drugs on the NCLEX-RN® will have generic names, remember that Trade names may differ in the US and Canada so it is wise to always learn the generic name. Generic names will also provide you with clues in regards to varying drug classes)**

Mechanism of Action: Loop-diuretic, acts in the proximal Loop of Henle, by blocking the reabsorption of sodium and chloride. This prevents the passive reabsorption of water. 20% of filtered NaCl is normally reabsorbed in this area of the kidney, therefore, significant diuresis occurs. **(knowing the mechanism of action will help you to predict differing side effects of medications)**

Therapeutic Uses: Rapid mobilization of fluid required for conditions such as: pulmonary edema associated with CHF, edema of hepatic, renal or cardiac origin, and hypertension not controlled with other diuretics. Useful in clients with severe renal impairment **(know the primary conditions the medication is used for so you can link the medication to different diseases or conditions in the exam questions)**

Excretion: Through the urine **(mechanisms of excretion will help you to determine risk of drug toxicity in cases of liver or renal failure, or if cytotoxic precautions are necessary)**

Protein Binding: 95% bound to plasma proteins **(drugs that are highly protein bound—i.e., 99% of drug is bound to plasma and not bioavailable in the blood—have the potential to become toxic in the system if the client has decreased volumes of circulating blood proteins OR if another drug has the ability to "bump" the drug off or compete for protein binding. If you encounter a drug that is 99% protein bound, also list signs of toxicity of the drug on your drug card—in this case with furosemide it is not a large concern)**

Therapeutic Index: Low or High? Furosemide has a high therapeutic index (meaning it does not have a high risk of toxicity) **(Does the drug have a low therapeutic index? If so, be familiar with serum levels and signs of drug toxicity)**

Known Drug Interactions: Digoxin, aminoglycoside drugs (e.g., gentamicin) because of increased risk of ototoxicity, lithium (furosemide can cause it to accumulate to toxic levels) **(focus in on drug-to-drug interactions that can cause toxicity or life-threatening symptoms)**

Important and specific side effects related to the medication: (this will help you to anticipate potential areas for assessment and intervention regarding the drug on the exam)

1. Hypotension
2. Hypokalemia
3. Ototoxicity

Nursing Implications (3 main focuses): (outline areas that you think have the potential for application or critical thinking questions on the exam. Focus on nursing assessments and interventions specific to drug therapy)

Excessive dehydration can lead to thrombosis and embolism. Hypotension results from loss of water and smooth muscle relaxation. Serum potassium may fall below therapeutic levels (3.5 Meq/L). Risk of dehydration can be lowered by initiating therapy with low doses, adjusting the dose carefully, monitoring weight loss daily, and giving furosemide on an intermittent schedule.

Hazard Vallerand, A. & Sanoski, C.A. (2014). Davis's drug guide for nurses (14th ed). Philadelphia: F.A. Davis

Tips for Making Drug Cards

- **Make them yourself rather than use pre-made drug cards**. The process of organizing information and choosing what is important will help you to better remember and apply information to the exam. Using pre-made cards only encourages memorization and not understanding of key concepts.
- **Keep them neat and simple**. It may be helpful to type them out rather than write on cards.
- **Use pictures, mnemonics or case studies to help you remember key information**. It may be useful to write a three sentence summary of a client who is receiving the medication. What would your key findings include if the client was experiencing adverse effects?
- **Think about *WHY* drug-to-drug actions occur with the medication, rather than trying to memorize drugs that interact**. For example, furosemide and digoxin have the potential to interact. This is because furosemide can decrease potassium levels and digoxin toxicity and dysrhythmias can occur when potassium is low or high. Find the links between the drugs and ensure that you understand them.
- **Always link your drug cards to pathology.** It is helpful to create SUMMARY MAPS of different disease conditions. Attach all the relevant drug cards to the disease condition you are studying (for an example of a disease study map, see: rnstudyguides.ca). Think about drug therapy alongside your other nursing interventions and understand how the drug therapy augments treatment.

PRACTICE QUESTIONS

Question 1

A client has taken an increased dose of ASA (Aspirin), an acidic drug. Which of the following foods would alkalize the urinary pH so that drug would be excreted faster?

1. Glass of Milk
2. Eggs
3. Cranberries
4. Prunes

Question 2

Jorge, 47 years old, is admitted to a medical unit with Chronic Obstructive Pulmonary Disorder. He is currently malnourished and has a low serum albumin. What will happen to Jorge if he is given a drug that is highly protein bound?

1. Jorge's kidneys will excrete the drug at a faster rate.
2. Jorge will be at risk of experiencing toxic effects of the drug.
3. Nothing as serum globulin is more important than serum albumin.
4. Jorge will be at risk of experiencing decreased effectiveness of the drug.

Question 3

A client is taking phenytoin and morphine sulfate concurrently. What should the nurse assess for in this situation?

1. Increased sedation, decreased respirations
2. Emergence of seizure activity
3. Increased levels of pain
4. Nausea and vomiting

Question 4

When hepatic blood flow is decreased in the older adult, this often decreases biotransformation (metabolism) of drugs. This most likely results in:

1. No effect
2. Slower excretion of the drug
3. More rapid excretion of the drug
4. Increase in drug dose requirement

Question 5

Prior to administering medications, the student nurse reviews the therapeutic index. Which statement best reflects that the student understands the therapeutic index?

1. The student is able to identify interactions among each drug the client is receiving.
2. The student is able to determine if the clients are receiving safe doses of medications.
3. The student is able to determine if the physician prescribed the best drug for the client.
4. The student is able to identify the clients who will need to have serum blood levels monitored.

Question 6

A client who has been on long-term warfarin therapy has been started on aprepitant after receiving chemotherapy. What should the nurse teach the client regarding the potential interaction between these two medications?

1. To ensure frequent monitoring of the client's INR levels
2. To watch for bleeding of the gums
3. To ensure that their vomiting is controlled
4. To ensure they are adequately hydrated

Answers: Question 1(1), Question 2(2), Question 3(1), Question 4(2), Question 5(4), Question 6(1)

Study Strategy

This study guide differs from other resources because formal rationale is not provided for the answers. **You need to determine the appropriate rationale for the correct answers by accessing the information in the question that may have inhibited your ability to answer the question correctly.** It is helpful to ask the following questions:

- What is the question asking? What are key words in the question query?
- What information do I need to know to answer this question correctly?
- How did I select my answer?
- Why were the other answers incorrect?
- Was I missing a piece of content knowledge that inhibited how I answered the question? If so, what should I target in on and study?

REFERENCES

Adams, M.P, Holland, L.N & Bostwick, P.M. (2008). Pharmacology for nurses: A pathophysiologic approach (2nd ed). New Jersey: Prentice Hall.

Hazard Vallerand, A. & Sanoski, C.A. (2014). Davis's drug guide for nurses (14th ed). Philadelphia: F.A. Davis

Lea, M.,Rognan, S.E., Koristovic, R., Wyller, T.B & Molden, E. (2013). Severity & management of drug-drug interactions in acute geriatric patients. *Drugs & Aging, 30*(9), 721-727. doi 10.1007/540266-013-0091-4

Richards, J.S. (2013). Overview of herbal supplements. *Elite Continuing Education, 46*-72.

Rosenjack Burchum, J. & Rosenthal, L.D. (2016). *Lehne's pharmacology for nursing care* (9th edition). St. Louis: Elsevier.

Silvestri, L.A. (2014). *Saunders comprehensive review for the NCLEX-RN® examination*. St. Louis: Elsevier.

Module 2

Drugs Affecting the Respiratory System

TABLE OF CONTENTS

Introduction to the Transitioning to the NCLEX-RN® Pharmacology Guide: Drugs Affecting the Respiratory System

The breadth and detail of the knowledge required of pharmacological concepts often overwhelms new graduates when they are beginning their exam preparation. The purpose of this pharmacology study guide is to help you work through the vast amount of pharmacological knowledge required for the NCLEX-RN® in a systematic and purposeful way. This guide organizes content using the current NCLEX-RN® Test Plan activity statements and provides specific strategies to address pharmacological areas of review which may challenge new graduates. **This is the second of twelve modules.** This is a working guide, so while key information will be presented and organized for review, it is up to you to do the detailed work of content review by answering the questions and exercises in each section. You can expect to see drugs described by their generic names on the exam. Due to the differences in drug trade names between the United States of America, Canada and other countries you should study drugs according to their generic names and develop strategies for remembering them.

This module is part of a comprehensive pharmacology study guide focusing on specific areas which may challenge NCLEX-RN® candidates. This includes drug-to-drug interactions, specific adverse reactions due to drug therapy and the potential reactions associated with herbal therapy and conventional medications. The content will be focused on a systems approach and will direct you towards important information within each drug class.

Structure of the Module

This module begins with an overview of the differing drug classes for the respiratory system. Additional areas for review that are specialized or affect multiple systems will also be highlighted:

1. Review questions and selected exercises will be constructed for each drug class to help pull out key concepts such as adverse events/side effects, specific client teaching and drug to drug interactions.
2. A summary chart of the drug classes in each system or theme will be provided for you to use alongside your other practice question resources. As you move through practice questions, check off the specific medications you come across and if you require further review in each area. It is also helpful to make your own drug cards for specific medications. Keep the drug cards simple. Identify the drug class, the mechanism of action, two relevant (i.e., life threatening) or unique adverse effects that require monitoring and provide an outline for client teaching or specific nursing interventions for the medication.

Advice for Studying Pharmacological Content for the NCLEX-RN®

Always start with areas you are NOT familiar with. For example, if you spent the majority of your time as a final practicum student/or nurse on a cardiology unit do not start in the Vascular and Cardiac Medications Module. It is common for students/graduates to move to areas of comfort when they are studying because it decreases their anxiety. However, your efforts should be targeted on what you don't know. Each Module in this series has a summary table of drugs for each system. Highlight the drug classes that you are not familiar with and make it your priority to work through them. Do not spend time making drug cards for medications you already know. For example, most students are confident with furosemide administration and can critically think through concepts associated with the drug. Therefore, time does not need to be spent studying this medication. Only make drug cards for medications that are new to you. The review questions in this guide will direct you towards more detailed information pertaining to the medications you are familiar with and focus on potential content areas where exam questions may be asked.

This guide is set up using a **systems approach** for the following reasons: 1) most pharmacology textbooks use this approach to structure content so it will be easier to find the information you need to answer the review questions; 2) using a systems approach allows you to find commonalties in the side effects of drugs influencing a specific system, so you will see patterns arising as you work through this guide; and 3) a systems approach allows for the creation of overall drug summary tables, which will be included in each module of the guide and will provide you with a general sense of the medications you need to cover.

The following resources will aid you in answering questions posed in this guide. This includes:

1. **A pharmacology textbook.** This resource will contain more detailed information pertaining to drug classes and outline general nursing considerations for therapy. I have referenced a pharmacology textbook throughout the writing of this guide.
2. **A drug guide**. These are the guides commonly used for your clinical practice. These resources contain alphabetized drug information. Most importantly, they outline specific pharmacokinetic and pharmacodynamics properties of drugs. You will find information related to drug excretion, protein binding, and therapeutic index in these guides.
3. **An online drug repository** for more detailed information that may not be found in the two resources above. Sometimes it is difficult to find therapeutic index and protein binding for a drug. I have found the following website helpful for this: http://www.drugbank.ca/drugs

Module 2: Drugs Affecting the Respiratory System

This module highlights common medications given for the respiratory system. These medications are addressed via their pharmacological classes. **It is important that you always study medications in the context of disease management/pathology**. Therefore, it is helpful if you also create strategies for studying medications alongside disease conditions. This module begins by condensing the different respiratory medication classes into a common table and listing specific medications. Then the remainder of the module contains review questions to help direct you to important information regarding each medication class. Exercises and strategies for approaching content in an exam context will be provided. You may find that the questions focus on more detailed information. The reason for this is to direct you away from studying common themes regarding these medications to more specific aspects of administration and monitoring.

Remember that management of the respiratory system is focused on maintaining the airway (upper and lower), decreasing inflammation, ensuring perfusion between the lungs and pulmonary system, and ensuring the body is not in a state of hypoxemia.

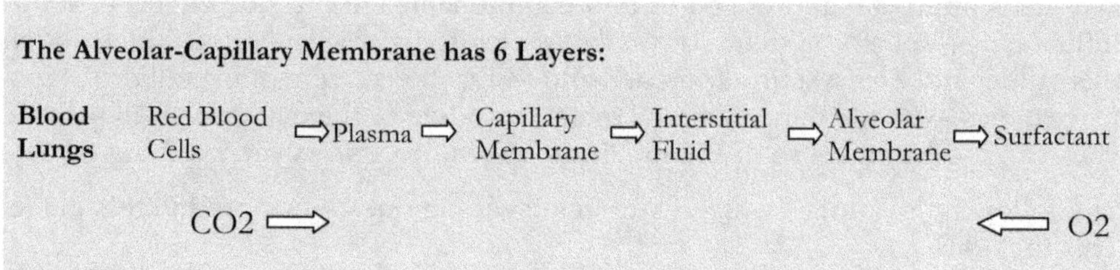

Copstead, L.E & Banaski, J. (2013). Pathophysiology (5th ed). St. Louis: Elsevier.

There are **four primary reasons** that a client would experience **hypoxemia** in the context of respiratory disease/failure (Copstead et al., 2013):

1. **Hypoventilation:** decreases in breaths/minute result in decreased oxygen and increased carbon dioxide levels
2. **Diffusion disturbances**: any pathology that causes the alveoli to fill with fluid (e.g., pneumonia), collapse (e.g., atelectasis)or decrease the surface area within the alveoli. More specifically, any condition that inhibits or slows the exchange of oxygen and carbon dioxide between the alveoli and pulmonary system. Other conditions, such as pulmonary fibrosis, cause the membrane between the alveoli and pulmonary system to become thickened and thereby cause delay in the diffusion of oxygen and carbon dioxide. This results in systemic hypoxia and hypercapnia.

3. **Shunting**: the process of shunting occurs when deoxygenated blood enters the pulmonary system and is not fully re-oxygenated to normal levels. Therefore, deoxygenated blood returns to the left side of the heart and is pumped out systemically. This results in systemic hypoxemia. This occurs in conditions such as pneumonia and ARDS.
4. **V/Q perfusion mismatch**: in this case ventilation and perfusion of oxygen are not equal. Causes are similar to the other indications for hypoxemia identified above (e.g. pneumonia, pulmonary edema, atelectasis).

Exercise 4

Create a list of common respiratory pathologies and ensure that you include classes of respiratory medications used to treat each condition. Identify any commonalities in the medications used for each condition. Ensure you are linking the mechanism of action of the medications with the pathophysiology of the condition.

Examples include:

- Chronic Obstructive Pulmonary Disorder
- Asthma
- Pneumonia
- Pulmonary Edema
- Pleural Effusion
- Pulmonary Fibrosis
- Influenza
- Sinusitis
- Tuberculosis
- Cystic Fibrosis

Table 2.1: Common Classes of Respiratory Medications

ANTIHISTAMINES	DECONGESTANTS	ANTITUSSIVES
Oral Chlorpheniramine Diphenhydramine Cetirizine Levocetirizine Fexofenadine Loratadine Desloratadine **Intranasal Antihistamines** Azelastine Olopatadine H1 receptors (smooth muscle contraction) H2 receptors (accelerate HR & gastric acid secretion)—see GI section Antihistamines compete directly with histamine for receptor sites H1 Blockers-diphenhydramine, tx of allergies, produce drowsiness, drying of mucous membranes Non-sedating: loratadine, cetirizine, fexofenadine	3 groups: 1. **Adrenergics (sympathomimetics):** ephedrine, phenylephrine, pseudoephedrine, naphazoline, oxymetazoline, terahydrozoline, xylometazoline 2. **Anticholinergics (parasympathomimetics)**: ipratropium nasal spray 3. **Topical corticosteroids combined with antihistamine:** azelastine/ fluticasone propionate This class is generally well-tolerated can cause nervousness, insomnia, palpations, tremor, mucosal irritation, dryness Excessive doses can cause increased levels in bloodstream resulting in alpha & beta stimulation.	Codeine Hydrocodone Dextromethorphan Diphenhydramine Benzonatate **2 categories** 1. **Opioid**—all have antitussive effects, but only codeine and hydrocodone are used for this purpose 2. **Non-opioid**—less effective: dextromethorphan

CORTICOSTERIODS	BETA$_2$-ADRENERGIC AGONISTS	ANTICHOLINERGICS
Inhaled Beclomethasone Budesonide Ciclesonide Flunisolide Fluticasone Mometasone **Oral** Methylprednisolone Prednisolone Prednisone Treatment of chronic inflammation for chronic asthma Do not relieve acute symptoms of asthma but are used to prevent an attack. Given by inhalation, orally, or IV in serve cases (beclomethasone, budesonide). Can cause pharyngeal irritation, coughing, dry mouth, oral fungal infections. These drugs have many interactions with other drugs.	**Inhaled, short acting** Albuterol Levalbuterol **Inhaled, Long Acting** Arformoterol Formoterol Indacaterol Salmeterol **Oral** Albuterol Terbutaline Acute phase of asthmatic attack. Agonists or stimulators of the SNS receptors (beta & alpha-adrenergic receptors- imitate effects of norepinephrine on receptors. To dilate airways Beta 2 receptors in lungs must be stimulated. Categorized according to receptors they stimulate: 1. Non-selective adrenergic drugs (alpha, beta$_1$, beta$_2$)—e.g., epinephrine 2. Non-selective beta-adrenergic drugs (beta$_1$, beta$_2$)—e.g., isoproterenol Selective (beta$_2$)—e.g., Ventolin **Noted side effects**: tachycardia, dysrhythmias, hypokalemia, hyperglycemia	Ipratropium Tiotropium Aclidinium Only anticholinergic typically used is ipratropium bromide- it is usually combined with beta2-agonist or fenoterol. No drugs are known to interact with ipratropium bromide. Used for prevention of bronchospasm associated with chronic bronchitis or emphysema, but is not for the management of acute symptoms.

XANTHINE DERIVATIVES/ METHYLXANTHINES	ANTILEUKOTRIENE AGENTS/ LEUKOTRIENE MODIFERS	EXPECTORANTS
Theophylline (Theo-Dur) Aminophylline (Truphylline)	Motelukast Zileuton Zafirlukast	Guaifenesin Iodinated glycerol Potassium iodide
Noted side effects: tachycardia, dysrhythmias, hypotension, seizures, circulatory failure, respiratory arrest	Combats immune cases of asthma. Leukotrienes cause inflammation, bronchoconstriction and mucus production, leading to coughing, wheezing & shortness of breath. Montelukast, Zafirlukast block actions of leukotrienes	Aid in coughing and expectoration of sputum Works by: 1. Reflex stimulation 2. Direction stimulation of secretory glands

REVIEW QUESTIONS

Drugs Focused on the Treatment of Asthma and COPD

Drugs for the treatment of COPD and asthma primarily fall into one of two categories: 1) bronchodilators or 2) anti-inflammatory medications. There are also anti-inflammatory/bronchodilator combinations.

Concepts for review:

1. Review how drugs are administered via inhalation and review pertinent client teaching: metered-dose inhalers, Respimats, dry-powder inhalers and nebulizers.
2. Outline the stepwise approach to the management of asthma. Identify which drug classes are used in each step.

BETA- AGONISTS

Beta-adrenergic agonists are a class of medications also referred to as bronchodilators and are used in the treatment of acute bronchospasm. They relax bronchial muscle resulting in a wider airway and increased ease of breath. It is important to remember that these medications do NOT have anti-inflammatory actions.

Beta-adrenergic agonists are best classified by their duration of action:

Drug Name	Duration of Action
Isoproterenol (Isuprel)	Ultrashort effects: 2-3 hours
Isoetharine (Bronkosol)	Ultrashort effects: 2-3 hours
Metaproterenol (Metaprel)	Short-acting effects: 5-6 hours
Terbutaline (Brethine)	Short-acting effects: 5-6 hours
Pirbuterol (Maxair)	Short-acting effects: 5-6 hours
Albuterol (Proventil)	Intermediate acting effects: 8 hours
Levalbuterol (Xopenex)	Intermediate acting effects: 8 hours
Bitolterol (Tornate)	Intermediate acting effects: 8 hours
Salmeterol (Serevent)	Long-acting effects: lasting as long as 12 hours
Formoterol (Foradil)	Combines rapid onset of action (1-3 min) with 12 hours duration

1. Determine if these medications have effects on Beta$_1$ and Beta$_2$ receptors or both. Outline side effects of the stimulation of Beta$_1$ receptors.

Tips for answering exam questions related to these medications (Rosenjack Burchum et al., 2016):

- Be able to differentiate between beta$_1$ and beta$_2$-receptors and note the importance of why beta$_2$ should be activated with these medications
- Understand the effects of beta$_2$ stimulation and why it treats asthma
- Ultrashort, short and intermediate acting bronchodilators are used to terminate acute asthmatic episodes
- Salmeterol's onset of action is too long to be indicated for asthma termination—it is given as a long acting bronchodilator
- Chronic use of these medications may cause tolerance and the dose may need to be increased or a second drug (glucocorticoid) may need to be introduced
- Increased used of these medications over a period of hours or days means that the client's condition is rapidly deteriorating and medical attention should be sought immediately
- Client teaching includes: limiting products that may contain caffeine, awareness that saliva and sputum may be pink after inhaler use
- If the question identifies symptoms of difficulty breathing, heart palpitations, tremors, vomiting, nervousness or vision changes, they need to be reported to the physician

- Instructions for the correct use of inhalers containing these medications include: having the client hold their breath for 10 seconds, waiting 2 minutes before the second inhalation and rinsing their mouth after use
- Note that Ventolin is called albuterol and salbutamol in different resources

Potential Drug-to-Drug Interactions

Non-selective beta blocker therapy will antagonize bronchodilation: use with caution with medications such as propranolol
MAO Inhibitors should be avoided because they will cause hypertension.
Persons with diabetes may require adjustments in their hypoglycemic agents because drugs such as epinephrine can increase blood glucose levels (Rosenjack Burchum et al., 2016).

Pediatric Considerations (Hockenberry & Wilson, 2010)

Bronchodilators, while used in pediatric populations, should be used with EXTREME CAUTION. Monitor for the following adverse effects: tremors, restlessness, GI tract upset, hallucinations, dizziness, palpitations, and tachycardia.
Common drugs administered to this population include: albuterol, metaproterenol and terbutaline for treatment of acute exacerbations of asthma and for prevention of exercise-induced bronchospasm. These medications should not be taken more than 3-4x per day. Salmeterol (Serevent) is a long-acting bronchodilator given twice a day.

Helpful Resource:

Canadian Thoracic Society (2010). 2010 CTS commentary on long-acting beta-2 agonist use for asthma in Canada. Author. Retrieved from http://www.respiratoryguidelines.ca/cts-commentary-laba-asthma

ANTICHOLINERGICS

Blocking the parasympathetic nervous system has similar effects to those caused by the sympathetic nervous system. Anticholinergic drugs cause bronchodilation. However, they should not be used in isolation to terminate an acute asthma attack. What are the benefits of combining anticholinergic medications with inhaled beta-agonists? (Two examples of combined drugs are: Combivent- ipratropium & albuterol).

1. What is Tiotropium (Spiriva) and what are its uses for COPD?
2. Which client populations are anticholinergic drugs NOT recommended for? (age parameters in particular).

3. The following assessments must be completed prior to administering anticholinergic drugs. Give rationale for each assessment:

Assessment focus	Rationale for assessment based on pharmacological effects of anticholinergic medications
Monitor vital signs, oxygen saturation, especially respiratory rate and pulse	
Assess respiratory effort, skin colour and lung sounds	
Assess for history of narrow-angle glaucoma	
Assess for history of benign prostatic hyperplasia	
Assess for history of renal disorders	
Assess for urinary bladder neck obstruction	

Tips for answering exam questions related to these medications (Rosenjack Burchum et al., 2016):

- They are never used to terminate an acute asthma attack
- They have a bitter taste, so encourage client to rinse their mouth
- Common adverse effects are related to changes in urinary patterns
- Anticholinergic crisis can occur from over-dosage: fever, tachycardia, difficulty swallowing, ataxia, reduced urine output, psychomotor agitation, confusion, and hallucinations
- Watch for side effects such as dysrhythmias and increased heart rate

METHYLXANTHINES

This group of bronchodilators is chemically related to caffeine (Rosenjack Burchum et al., 2016, p.928). The two most common drugs are theophylline and aminophylline.

1. Theophylline has a very narrow margin of safety. Why? What should the nurse assess for when administering this medication?

2. Why are these medications contraindicated in clients with angina pectoris or coronary artery disease?
3. What are serious adverse effects occurring with these medications?
4. How does tobacco and marijuana smoke influence theophylline metabolism?

Tips for answering exam questions related to these medications (Rosenjack Burchum et al., 2016):

- In questions focused on nutrition/diet and methylxanthines, remember that you are to limit the use of products containing caffeine
- Early signs of toxicity are: anorexia, nausea, vomiting, dizziness, restlessness, hypotension or seizures
- Cigarette smoking reduces the therapeutic response of these medications
- OTC cold medications should not be taken without notifying a healthcare provider
- Lab testing is required because of narrow safety margins
- Rifampin, phenobarbital and phenytoin can lower theophylline levels—concurrent use of these medications may require an increase in theophylline dose
- Theophylline is given orally or by IV. Doses are based on weight and age and increased slowly. IV theophylline is reserved for emergencies and is administered slowly
- Aminophylline is given IV and Orally. IV loading dose is 6mg/kg and, like theophylline, infused slowly
- Adult therapeutic range for theophylline is 5-15 mcg/mL
- Adult therapeutic range for aminophylline is 10-20 mcg/mL

Pediatric Considerations (Hockenberry et al., 2010)

Theophylline is considered a third line agent for pediatric management and unnecessary for treating asthma exacerbations. When it is used in children, serum concentrations must be monitored (same in adults). Therapeutic effects are between 5-15 mcg/mL. Maximum levels of 15 mcg/mL are recommended for outpatient care.

Toxicity can occur with levels 20 mcg/mL or greater. Early signs of toxicity are nausea, tachycardia, irritability
Severe toxicity occurs with levels 30 mcg/mL or greater. Signs are seizures and dysrhythmias.

INHALED GLUCOCORTICOIDS

Glucocorticoids dampen the activation of the inflammatory response by producing anti-inflammatory mediators and making the bronchial smooth muscle more responsive to beta-agonist stimulation. They are administered systemically and by inhalation. Their primary purpose is to prevent an asthma attack, not to treat an acute attack. This section will focus on inhaled glucocorticoids in the context of asthma and COPD. However, for severe unstable asthma clients may be put on oral prednisone for 5-7 days and then switched to inhaled glucocorticoids (Rosenjack Burchum et al., 2016, p.923).

1. Why would determining FEV_1 as well as frequency and severity of asthma attacks be recommended prior to prescribing glucocorticoid therapy?
2. Can clients with a positive sputum culture for Candida albicans receive inhaled glucocorticoids?
3. Why is alternate every other day dosing recommended for oral dosing of glucocorticoids?
4. Why must clients who have switched from long-term oral glucocorticoids to inhaled glucocorticoids take supplemental systemic glucocorticoids at times of severe stress?
5. What should the nurse teach clients regarding the prevention of bone loss when taking this class of medications?

Tips for answering exam questions related to these medications (Rosenjack Burchum et al., 2016):

- Infection can result from these medications—pay attention to any changes in vital signs or increases in temperature
- Blood glucose monitoring is important for people with diabetes
- Assess for any signs tarry stools, edema, dizziness or difficulty breathing
- Medications are not used for terminating acute asthma attacks (use a beta-agonist)
- Rinse mouth after use
- Potassium losses can occur—diet focused questions related to glucocorticoid therapy should focus on adding potassium rich foods and monitoring for hypokalemia
- Aspirin is not to be used—clients should notify their healthcare provider if they are taking ASA
- Dosing should be consistent—clients are not to adjust their dose independently, omit doses or change intervals between dosing
- Always pay attention to the question and note if the glucocorticoid is being given via inhalation (minimal systemic side effects) or systemically via oral dosage (maximum systemic side effects will occur).
- Clients on prolonged systemic glucocorticoid therapy will experience a decrease in production of endogenous production of glucocorticoids by the adrenal glands. If oral therapy is stopped suddenly, the client can die; if the client is in a stress state (e.g., involved in an accident and in hospital) and the glucocorticoid dose is not increased, they can also die. Switching from oral glucocorticoids to inhaled glucocorticoids must be done slowly to allow the body to resume producing its own hormones via the adrenal glands.

- During times of extreme stress client on glucocorticoid therapy via inhalation or oral administration must be given supplemental oral or IV glucocorticoid therapy.

Pediatric Considerations

There is strong evidence that inhaled steroids improve long term outcomes in children of all ages with mild to moderate persistent asthma. Inhaled corticosteroids at recommended doses do not have long-term, significant effects on growth, bone mineral density, ocular toxicity, or suppression of adrenal/pituitary axis (Hockenberry et al., 2010).
Nurses and Health Care Providers should monitor growth frequently (q3-6 months) to assess for any systemic effects of these drugs and make reductions of doses as necessary.

LEUKOTRIENE MODIFIERS

Leukotrienes are chemical mediators of inflammation that cause edema, inflammation, and bronchoconstriction when released. Drugs in this class work in one of two ways. The first is by blocking lipoxygenase, an enzyme that synthesizes leukotrienes (e.g., zileuton [Zyflo]), and the second is by blocking leukotriene receptors (e.g., zarfirlukast (Accolate) and montelukast (Singulair). The key action of these medications is the reduction of inflammation—they do indirectly reduce bronchoconstriction, but are not considered bronchodilators like beta-agonists. These medications are given orally (Rosenjack Burchum et al., 2016, p.924-925).

1. What neuropsychiatric effects are often associated with drugs in this medication class?
2. Are these drugs given as first- or second-line medications?
3. Which lab test should be conductedregularly in clients receiving zileuton?
4. What do zileuton and zafirlukast do to drugs such as warfarin, theophylline and propranolol? (hint: increase or decrease levels of these drugs)
5. Churg-Strauss Syndrome is associated with the administration of zafirlukast and montelukast. What are the symptoms of this syndrome? (concurrent glucocorticoid withdrawal with the administration of zafirlukast is thought to increase the changes of this syndrome)
6. What are the 3 indications for the administration of montelukast?

Tips for answering exam questions related to these medications (Rosenjack Burchum et al., 2016):

- There is an increased risk of infection in persons older than 65 years of age when using these medications
- Side effects to report immediately are: nausea, fatigue, lethargy, itching, abdominal pain, dark-coloured urine and flulike symptoms

- Be aware of pre-existing hepatic failure—these clients shouldn't take this class of medication
- If a client is on warfarin, closely monitor prothrombin time (PT) and international normalized ratio (INR) in clients concurrently taking coumadin
- Monitor phenytoin level with concurrent phenytoin therapy
- Reduce theophylline dose and monitor levels (zileuton) if client is using this therapy concurrently
- Closely monitor heart rate and blood pressure in clients taking propranolol (Inderal)
- Monitor effectiveness of montelukast in clients taking phenobarbital concurrently
- Omalizumab forms complexes with free IgE antibodies in the blood and prevents the activation of mast cells, it is administered sc and peak plasma levels take 7-8 days (only helps clients whose asthma is triggered by certain allergens)

Pediatric Considerations

Omalizumab (Xolair) is the only drug approved by the FDA for the treatment of asthma in children greater than 12 years of age. This drugs blocks IgE from binding to Mast Cells and is administered once or twice a month by sc injection.

MAST CELL STABILIZERS

These drugs are focused on inhibiting mast cells from releasing histamine and other chemical mediators of inflammation (p.925).

1. Cromolyn (Intal) is administered via MDI or nebulizer. What are side effects of this medication and how often should it be dosed?
2. Nedocromil (Tilade) has a longer half-life than cromolyn (Intal) and similar side effects. Which side effect, in particular, is responsible for clients discontinuing therapy?

Tips for answering exam questions related to these medications (Rosenjack Burchum et al., 2016):

- Cromolyn is administered as a powder-driven nebulizer and is the safest of all anti-asthma medications
- Cromolyn is indicated for chronic asthma, exercise-induced bronchospasm and allergic rhinitis

Other Respiratory Medications:

SYMPATHOMIMETICS (DECONGESTANTS)

These drugs reduce nasal congestion by activating alpha$_1$-adrenergic receptors on nasal blood vessels, this causes vasoconstriction and shrinkage of swollen membranes followed by nasal drainage. Topical administration is rapid and intense, while oral administration responses may be delayed, moderate or prolonged (Rosenjack Burchum et al., 2016, p.941).

1. What are common adverse effects with this classification of medications?
2. How long should topical sympathomimetics be used for?
3. How should sympathomimetics in drop form be administered?
4. What is the difference between phenylephrine, ephedrine and pseudoephedrine?

ANTITUSSIVES

These drugs are used to treat dry hacking non-productive coughs in order to reduce irritation of the throat and to allow the client to rest. These medications should only be used if the cough is interfering with activities of daily living, rest or sleep (Rosenjack Burchum et al., 2016, p.944).

Drug	Adverse Effects
Opioid Antitussives: - codeine - hydrocodone bitartrate (Hycodan)	Severe: hypotension, seizures, bradycardia, respiratory depression, severe somnolence
Non-Opioid Antitussives: - benzonatate (Tessalon)	Severe: paradoxical excitation, tremors, euphoria, insomnia
- dextromethorphan (Benylin)	Severe: CNS depression, paradoxical excitation Allow chemically similar to codeine, it does not cause dependence

1. Which client populations should these drugs NOT be used for? What precautions should be taken in clients with chronic lung disease?
2. How to opioids work to depress the cough reflex?
3. How does benzonatate work to suppress the cough reflex? What happens if the pill is chewed by the client?

Tips for answering exam questions related to these medications (Rosenjack Burchum et al., 2016):

- Report any changes in the colour of sputum especially if it is yellow or green tinged
- If taking a prescriptive antitussive medication (this is typically the opioid antitussives) teach the client not to take OTC cough preparations without notifying the health care provider, they may cause excessive drowsiness
- Teach clients taking opioid antitussives to avoid driving or performing hazardous activities and to avoid alcohol use.
- Store opioid antitussives away from children
- Benzonatate can cause numbness in the mouth and throat if chewed
- Dextromethorphan (Benylin) can cause CNS depression—assess for signs of this response in clients taking this therapy
- Opioid antitussive drugs can cause hypotension, seizures, bradycardia, respiratory depression and severe somnolence—in these cases the client can be treated with naloxone (Narcan)
- Drugs that can potentiate CNS depression in opioid antitussive medications include: other opioid medications, antihistamines, antipsychotics, antianxiety agents, alcohol. If combined therapy is indicated (e.g., hydrocodone bitartrate and an antihistamine), the dose of one or both drugs should be reduced.
- Hydrocodone bitartrate may increase the effect of MAO inhibitors and tricyclicantidepressants

ANTIHISTAMINES

In this context, antihistamines are only used for allergic rhinitis.

1. Identify common first-generation (sedating) oral antihistamines.
2. Identify common second-generation (non-sedating) oral antihistamines.
3. There are two common intranasal antihistamines, azelastine (Astelin) and olopatadine (Patanase), that are given to adults and children over the age of 12. What can systemic absorption of these drugs cause?
4. Which antihistamine drugs are safe to give to children: a) under 10kg, and b) 6-11 years of age, and c) over 12 years of age?

EXPECTORANTS AND MUCOLYTICS

Expectorants increase bronchial secretions and mucolytics help loosen thick bronchial secretions so secretions can be removed more easily by coughing. Common drugs include:

Guaifenesin (Robitussin) = expectorant

Acetylcysteine (Mucomyst) = mucolytic

BEST PRACTICE GUIDELINES

Best practice guidelines can help you to structure your study approach to disease management. Use the following guidelines below to help you prioritize key nursing interventions and to focus in on medical management of varying respiratory conditions.

Canadian Thoracic Society (2010). 2010 CTS commentary on long-acting beta-2 agonist use for asthma in Canada. Author. Retrieved from http://www.respiratoryguidelines.ca/cts-commentary-laba-asthma

Registered Nurses' Association of Ontario (2004). Adult asthma care guidelines for nurses: Promoting control of asthma. Retrieved from http://rnao.ca/bpg/guidelines/adult-asthma-care-guidelines-nurses-promoting-control-asthma

Registered Nurses' Association of Ontario (March, 2004). *The goal is asthma control.*Toronto: Author. Retrieved from http://rnao.ca/bpg/fact-sheets/goal-asthma-control

Registered Nurses' Association of Ontario (December, 2005). *Chronic obstructive pulmonary disease (COPD): Helping you breathe easier.* Toronto: Author. Retrieved from http://rnao.ca/bpg/fact-sheets/chronic-obstructive-pulmonary-disease-copd-%E2%80%93-helping-you-breathe-better

Registered Nurses' Association of Ontario (2005). Nursing care of Dyspnea: The 6th vital sign in individuals with chronic obstructive pulmonary disease. Toronto: Author. Retrieved from http://rnao.ca/bpg/guidelines/dyspnea

Qaseem, A., Wilt, T.J.,Winberger, S.E., Hanania, N.A., Criner, G., van der Molen, T....Shekelle, P. (2011). Diagnosis and management of stable chronic obstructive pulmonary disease: A clinical practice guideline update from the American college of physicians, American college of chest physicians, American thoracic society, and European respiratory society. *ACP Clinical Practice Guidelines, Annals of Internal Medicine,* 155,179-191. Retrieved from https://www.thoracic.org/statements/resources/copd/179full.pdf

PRACTICE QUESTIONS

Question 1

A client has been admitted with an acute asthmatic episode. List in order of priority the following medications to be given to the client.

1. prednisone	1.
2. albuterol	2.
3. theophylline	3.
4. salmeterol	4.

Question 2

A client is receiving aminophylline orally. Which of the following foods should the client be taught to avoid when taking this medication? **Select all that apply**:

1. Fermented foods and cheese
2. Coffee
3. Black Tea
4. Bananas
5. Energy drinks

Question 3

A child with persistent asthma is receiving theophylline therapy. On assessment, the child demonstrates nausea, tachycardia and irritability. What should the nurse anticipate the serum theophylline level to be on the bloodwork?

1. 5-10 mcg/mL
2. 10-15 mcg/mL
3. 20 mcg/mL
4. 30mcg/mL or greater

Question 4

A client who was on long-term oral glucocorticoid therapy has had the therapy discontinued and was recently started on inhaled glucocorticoid therapy. What is a critical factor the nurse must teach for a client who has had this specific change in therapy?

1. The client should avoid public spaces to prevent infection.
2. The client should keep extra oral glucocorticoid medications for times of extreme stress or illness.
3. The client should monitor their blood glucose levels daily.
4. The client should use this therapy for acute asthma attacks.

Question 5

A client is receiving Zileuton and propranolol at the same time. What should the nurse assess for in regards to combining the administration of these medications?

1. Recurrent tachycardia
2. Prolonged bleeding
3. Bronchospasm
4. Increased inflammation of the airways

Question 6

A confused client chews a benzonatate pill when the nurse administers the medication instead of swallowing it. What is a priority nursing intervention in this situation?

1. Observe for increased effects of the medication
2. Offer water or juice to the client to rid the bitter taste in their mouth
3. Assess for increased drowsiness and decreased level of consciousness
4. Observe for throat numbness and impaired ability to swallow

Answers: Question 1 (albuterol, salmeterol, theophylline, prednisone), Question 2: coffee, black tea, energy drink (all contain caffeine), Question 3(3), Question 4(2), Question 5(1), Question 6(4)

Study Strategy

This study guide differs from other resources because formal rationale is not provided for the answers. **You need to determine the appropriate rationale for the correct answers by accessing the information in the question that may have inhibited your ability to answer the question correctly**. It is helpful to ask the following questions:

- What is the question asking? What are key words in the question query?
- What information do I need to know to answer this question correctly?
- How did I select my answer?
- Why were the other answers incorrect?
- Was I missing a piece of content knowledge that inhibited how I answered the question? If so, what should I target in on and study?

Additional Strategies for Working with the Pharmacology Study Guide Modules

Content review is essential for being successful at answering NCLEX-RN® exam questions focusing on pharmacology. The following tips will help you to navigate the breath of this content and to organize your study notes.**Remember that you need to do the work of solid content review in order to be successful in understanding pharmacological concepts. Do not rely on practice questions to teach you what you need to know regarding medications for the NCLEX-RN®- practice questions are a tool for consolidating knowledge not a primary way to study.**

1. Complete the exercises in this study guide and make notes. This guide has been designed to direct you to important content for medication review. When creating the study guide I used an educator's lens to pull out the most important information in order ensure client safety with drug administration. For example, when review differing drugs I focused on critical information and essential education for each drug. The review questions are designed to bring this information forward.
2. Find ways to colour code or organize medications according to the bodily system or pathology they are used for. This will help you with recalling information. This guide uses a systems approach to help you organize the vast amount of pharmacological review in a way that will help you understand key concepts and pathologies.
3. Create case studies or unique ways to remember classes of medications. It is always wise to study pharmacology in the context of pathology. Use case studies specifically for content that is new to you or more difficult. Case studies should be memorable, contain client information that is easy to remember, focus on adverse effects of medications and key aspects of client education.

4. It is helpful to find patterns in names in drugs- such as suffixes that are common. Highlight the endings of common terms and find strategies to remember the main side effects of these classes of medications.
5. Client teaching is essential in medication administration. Ensure that you review your client education chapter in your Fundamentals of Nursing text-book (e.g. Potter and Perry). You need to remember that the use of basic teaching and learning principles paired with your knowledge of medica-tions can help you to better exam questions.
6. When you use practice questions find consistent strategies for reviewing questions that you get incorrect. For example, the summary drug tables presented in each module of this guide provide a structure for organizing information. Create a blank table with the drug classes named for each sys-tem. Write information or content that is tested in each drug class as you move through your practice resources. Highlight the medication names you have seen in the practice questions on your summary table. Are there any patterns in the types of questions asked or the content tested? **Do be care-ful with this strategy- it is not a replacement for reviewing content.**

Conclusion

Strong pharmacological review will not only increase your chances of success on the NCLEX-RN® it will also strengthen your future nursing practice. The com-plexity of client care paired with the increase in co-morbidity and chronic disease management poses many challenges to pharmacological therapy. Nurses must be aware of potential drug-to-drug interactions, polypharmacy, and adverse events related to medications in order to keep their clients safe. I wish you all the best for your NCLEX-RN® exam and for your future nursing practice.

Best wishes,

Dr. Marnie Kramer-Kile

REFERENCES

Copstead, L.E & Banaski, J. (2013). *Pathophysiology* (5th ed). St. Louis: Elsevier.

Richards, J.S. (2013). Overview of herbal supplements. *Elite Continuing Education*, 46-72.

Rosenjack Burchum, J. & Rosenthal, L.D. (2016). *Lehne's pharmacology for nursing care* (9th edition). St. Louis: Elsevier.

Module 3

Drugs Affecting the Nervous System

TABLE OF CONTENTS

Tables and Figures

Introduction to the Transitioning to the NCLEX-RN® Pharmacology Guide: Drugs Affecting the Nervous System

The breadth and detail of the knowledge required of pharmacological concepts often overwhelms new graduates when they are beginning their exam preparation. The purpose of this pharmacology study guide is to help you work through the vast amount of pharmacological knowledge required for the NCLEX-RN® in a systematic and purposeful way. This guide organizes content using the current NCLEX-RN® Test Plan and provides specific strategies to address pharmacological areas of review which may challenge new graduates. **This is the third of twelve modules.** This is a working guide, so while key information will be presented and organized for review, it is up to you to do the detailed work of content review by answering the questions and exercises in each section. You can expect to see drugs described by their generic names on the exam. Due to the differences in drug trade names between the United States of America, Canada and other countries you should study drugs according to their generic names and develop strategies for remembering them.

This module is part of a comprehensive pharmacology study guide focusing on specific areas which may challenge NCLEX-RN® candidates. This includes drug-to-drug interactions, specific adverse reactions due to drug therapy and the potential reactions associated with herbal therapy and conventional medications. The content will be focused on a systems approach and will direct you towards important information within each drug class.

Structure of the Module

This module begins with an overview of the differing drug classes for the nervous system. Additional areas for review that are specialized or affect multiple systems will also be highlighted:

1. Review questions and selected exercises will be constructed for each drug class to help pull out key concepts such as adverse events/side effects, specific client teaching and drug to drug interactions.
2. A summary chart of the drug classes in each system or theme will be provided for you to use alongside practice questions. As you move through practice questions, check off the specific medications you come across and if you require further review in each area. It is also helpful to make your own drug cards for specific medications. Keep the drug cards simple. Identify the drug class, the mechanism of action, two relevant (i.e., life threatening) or unique adverse effects that require monitoring and provide an outline for client teaching or specific nursing interventions for the medication.

Advice for Studying Pharmacological Content for the NCLEX-RN®

Always start with areas you are NOT familiar with. For example, if you spent the majority of your time as a final practicum student/or nurse on a cardiology unit do not start in the Vascular and Cardiac Medications Module. It is common for students/graduates to move to areas of comfort when they are studying because it decreases their anxiety. However, your efforts should be targeted on what you don't know. Each Module in this series has a summary table of drugs for each system. Highlight the drug classes that you are not familiar with and make it your priority to work through them. Do not spend time making drug cards for medications you already know. For example, most students are confident with furosemide administration and can critically think through concepts associated with the drug. Therefore, time does not need to be spent studying this medication. Only make drug cards for medications that are new to you. The review questions in this guide will direct you towards more detailed information of the medications that you are familiar with and focus on potential areas where exam questions may be asked.

This guide is set up using a **systems approach** for the following reasons: 1) most pharmacology textbooks use this approach to structure content so it will be easier to find the information you need to answer the review questions; 2) using a systems approach allows you to find commonalties in the side effects of drugs influencing a specific system, so you will see patterns arising as you work through this guide; and 3) a systems approach allows for the creation of overall drug summary tables, which will be included in each module of the guide and will provide you with a general sense of the medications you need to cover.

The following resources will aid you in answering questions posed in this guide. This includes:

1. **A pharmacology textbook.** This resource will contain more detailed information pertaining to drug classes and outline general nursing considerations for therapy. I have referenced a pharmacology textbook throughout the writing of this guide.
2. **A drug guide**. These are the guides commonly used for your clinical practice. These resources contain alphabetized drug information. Most importantly, they outline specific pharmacokinetic and pharmacodynamics properties of drugs. You will find information related to drug excretion, protein binding, and therapeutic index in these guides.
3. **An online drug repository** for more detailed information that may not be found in the two resources above. Sometimes it is difficult to find therapeutic index and protein binding for a drug. I have found the following website helpful for this: http://www.drugbank.ca/drugs

Module 3: Drugs Affecting the Nervous System

Neuropharmacologic agents act on one of two basic neuronal activities:

1. **Axonal conduction** (only a few drugs influence axonal conduction and this action is non-selective—local anesthetics do this)
2. **Synaptic transmission** (the majority of drugs influence synaptic transmission and the effects are more selective)

The focus in this module will primarily be on drugs influencing synaptic transmission. In order to understand this concept and how these medications work, it is important to review the basic steps in synaptic transmission. In order for a drug to impact a neuronally-regulated process, it must directly or indirectly influence receptor activity on the target cells (Rosenjack Burchum & Rosenthal., 2016, p. 97). Drugs will either **enhance** receptor activation or **reduce** receptor activation.

Table 3.1 Steps in Synaptic Transmission (Rosenjack Burchum et al., 2016, p. 97-98)

Step	What happens in this process	How Drugs Act in this Step
Step 1: Transmitter Synthesis	Molecules of transmitter must be present in the nerve terminal (molecules form in the presynaptic nerve terminal to make a transmitter [T])	Drugs can: 1. Increase transmitter synthesis (causes receptor activation to increase by increasing the amount of transmitter stored). 2. Decrease transmitter synthesis (causes receptor activation to decrease by decreasing the amount of transmitter stored). 3. Cause the synthesis of transmitter molecules that are more effective than the natural transmitter itself (causes receptor storage to increase).
Step 2: Transmitter Storage	Once the transmitter (T) is synthesized it is stored until it is released in the axon terminal. The transmitter is stored in tiny packets in the axon terminal.	Drugs can interfere with transmitter storage and cause receptor activation to decrease.

Step 3: Transmitter Release	The arrival of an action potential triggers the release of the transmitter (T) at the axon terminal. Only a small fraction of all vesicles present in the axon terminal discharge their contents.	Drugs can either promote or inhibit transmitter release. Drugs that promote release increase receptor activation. Drugs that inhibit release reduce receptor activation.
Step 4: Receptor Binding	Transmitter molecules diffuse across the synaptic gap and undergo reversible binding to receptors on the postsynaptic cell. This binding causes a cascade of events that result in altered behaviour on the postsynaptic cell.	Drugs can: 1. Bind to receptors and cause receptor activation (agonists—e.g., morphine on opiate receptors). 2. Bind to receptors and block receptor activation (antagonists—e.g., narcan on opiate receptors). 3. Bind to receptor components and enhance receptor activation by the natural transmitter at the site (e.g., benzodiazapines).
Step 5: Termination of Transmission	Transmission is terminated by dissociating the transmitter from its receptors and removing any free transmitter remaining in the synaptic gap.	Drugs interfere with the termination action by: 1. Blocking transmitter uptake. 2. Inhibiting transmitter degradation. In both these mechanisms, the goal of drug therapy is to increase transmitter availability and increase receptor activation.

In order to fully understand neuropharmacological therapy, you need to review the different neurotransmitters and receptors in both the CNS and PNS. The table below (Table 3.2) summarizes key neurotransmitters in each system. The most significant for your study are highlighted in red.

Table 3.2 Summary of Neurotransmitters in the Central and Peripheral Nervous System (Rosenjack Burchum et al., 2016, p. 105-110, 174)

Central Nervous System	Peripheral Nervous System
21 compounds serve as neurotransmitters (red highlights most common in drug therapy): **Monoamines:** Dopamine, Epinephrine, Norepinephrine, Serotonin **Amino Acids:** Aspartate, GABA, Glutamate, Glycine **Purines:** Adenosine, Adenosine monophosphate, Adenosine triphosphate **Opioid Peptides:** Dynorphins, Endorphins, Enkephalins **Nonopioid Peptides:** Neurotensin, Oxytocin, Somatostatin, Substance P, Vasopressin **Others**: Acetylcholine, Histamine **Blood/Brain Barrier**: **Only lipid-soluble drugs can cross; Protein-bound drugs and highly ionized drugs cannot cross.** It is not fully understood how CNS drugs act; only plausible hypothesis have been formed.	**Parasympathetic Nervous System**: Acetylcholine (various organs) **Sympathetic Nervous System**: Acetylcholine (various organs, sweat glands), epinephrine (various organs), norepinephrine (various organs) **Somatic Nervous System:** Acetylcholine *All preganglionic neurons release acetylcholine- postganglionic neurons, depending on nervous system, will release acetylcholine, norepinephrine or epinephrine.

REVIEW QUESTIONS

1. Complete the following tables in order to better understand the actions of receptors in the nervous system and their relation to drug therapy:

Adrenergic Receptor Type	Location in the Body	Action when Stimulated	Neurotransmitter Acting on Receptor
Alpha$_1$ Receptors			
Alpha$_2$ Receptors			
Beta$_1$ Receptors			

$Beta_2$ Receptors			
Dopamine Receptors			

Cholinergic Receptor Type	Location in the Body	Action when Stimulated	Neurotransmitter Acting on Receptor
$Nicotinic_N$			
$Nicotinic_M$			
Muscarinic			

REVIEW QUESTIONS

There are **six categories** of cholinergic drugs; an example of a prototype drug for review is presented for each class:

I. **Muscarinic agonists**: Bethanechol
II. **Muscarinic antagonists:** Atropine
III. **Ganglionic stimulation agents**: Nicotine
IV. **Ganglionic blocking agents**: Mecamylamine
V. **Neuromuscular blocking agents**: Succinylcholine, pancuronium, rocuronium (these drugs are given for rapid intubation, during surgery and in critical care areas—they are not covered in detail in this guide: I suggest you make drug cards for the three drugs identified above)
VI. **Cholinesterase inhibitors**: Neostigmine

Tips for Studying these Medications

1. Create a drug card for each of these medications and describe their indications for use.
2. Focus in on adverse effects of each of these medications and create a teaching plan to address them. Common adverse effects include: xerostomia, blurred vision, photophobia, urinary retention, constipation, hyperthermia, tachycardia.
3. What are signs of excessive muscarinic stimulation? How is this treated?
4. Why is atropine contraindicated for clients with glaucoma, intestinal atony, urinary tract obstruction, and tachycardia? (*This will help you to understand its mechanism of action and indications for use*).

Drug-to-Drug Interactions (Rosenjack Burchum et al., 2016)

Clients receiving atropine or other anticholinergic drugs can have excessive muscarinic blockade if they are also receiving: antihistamines, tricyclic antidepressants or phenothiazines.
Overdose of anticholinergic drugs (muscarinic poisoning) can mimic psychosis.
Treatment of overdose is typically the administration of activated charcoal for oral medications and physostigmine.

The remainder of this module will focus on pharmacological treatment for various neurological conditions. Table 3.3 contains a medication list for common neurological conditions and review questions will follow. It is always helpful to spend time reviewing the basic pathophysiology of each disease condition. This will help you to predict the mechanism of action of the drug and its potential adverse effects. The following resources provide additional information regarding some of the pathologies listed below:

Table 3.3 Drugs Affecting the Nervous System

Drugs for Epilepsy	**Drugs for Multiple Sclerosis**	**Drugs for Muscle Spasm and Spasticity**
Phenytoin Fosphenytoin Carbamazepine Valporic Acid Ethosuximide Phenobarbital Primidone Oxycarbazeine Lamotrigine Gabapentin Pregabalin Levetiracetam Topiramate Tiagabine Zonisamide Felbamate Lacosamide Rufinamide Vigabatrin Ezogabine	Interferon Beta: Interferon beta-1a, Interferon beta-1b Dimethyl furmate Glatiramer acetate Natalizumab Fingolimod Teriflunomide Mitoxantrone	Baclofen Diazepam Dantrolene **Drugs for Alzheimer's Disease** Cognitive Impairment Cholinesterase Inhibitors: donepezil, rivastigmine, galantamine Memantine
	Drugs for Parkinson's Disease Levodopa Levodopa/Carbidopa Dopamine Agonists (pramipexole, ropinirole, rotigotin, apomorphine, bromocriptine, cabergoline) COMT Inhibitors (entacapone) MAO-B Inhibitors (selegiline, amantadine)	**Drugs for Myasthenia Gravis** Neostigmine Physostigmine Donepezil Edrophonium Galantamine Pyridostigmine Rivastigmine

REVIEW QUESTIONS

MYASTHENIA GRAVIS

1. Cholinesterase inhibitors are used to treat this condition. What are contraindications for the administration of this class of medications?
   *Note that caution should be exercised in clients with: PUD, bradycardia, asthma or hyperthyroidism.
2. What would be signs of insufficient and excessive dosing of these types of medications?
3. What are signs of excessive muscarinic stimulation?
4. What is myasthenic crisis? What are the signs of this condition (this is an important concept).

Tips for answering exam questions related to these medications (Rosenjack Burchum et al., 2016):

- Dosing is contingent on the therapeutic response of the drug, teach clients to recognize effective dosing
- Physostigmine is the drug of choice for muscarinic antagonist poisoning (e.g., if too much atropine has been given)
- IV atropine can, in turn, alleviate muscarinic effects of cholinesterase inhibition (in drugs such as neostigmine)
- Excessive muscarinic stimulation is treated with atropine—ensure you can recognize the symptoms of this adverse effect
- Be able to differentiate cholinergic crisis (cholinesterase inhibitor overdose; skeletal muscle paralysis from neuromuscular blockade and signs of excessive muscarinic stimulation—salivation, sweating, miosis, bradycardia) from myasthenic crisis

PARKINSON'S DISEASE

1. Levodopa may be taken with food but high protein meals should be avoided. Why?
2. How long does it take for the client to feel the full benefits of Levodopa?
3. What happens when Levodopa is combined with a dopamine agonist (e.g., Pramixpexole), a COMT inhibitor (e.g., Entacapone) or an MAO-B inhibitor (e.g., Rasagline)?
4. Identify potential levodopa-induced movement disorders.
5. What would be signs of excessive cardiac stimulation for clients receiving Levodopa?
6. What is levodopa induced psychosis? What are symptoms of it? How is it treated?
7. Dopamine agonists (apomorphine, bromocriptine, cabergoline, pramipexole, rotigotin, ropinirole) cause similar side effects to those of Levodopa.

However, they may also induce sleep attacks. What are sleep attacks and what would the nurse teach the client regarding this potential side effect?
8. What should the nurse teach clients of child-bearing age about ropinirole?

Tips for answering exam questions related to these medications (Rosenjack Burchum et al., 2016)

- Sometimes these medications have an acute loss of effect—these "off" times can be reduced by combining levodopa/carbidopa with a dopamine agonist, a COMT inhibitor or MAO-B inhibitor
- High protein meals can cause "off" times, i.e., acute loss of effect of Levodopa/Carbidopa
- Tremors, dystonic movements and twitching are signs of dyskinesia—stop Leveodopa/Carbidopa and call HCP to reduce dosage
- Watch for signs of excessive cardiac stimulation with Levodopa/Carbidopa
- Levodopa-induced psychosis can occur—this condition is often treated with clozapine or quetiapine
- Apomorphine is reserved for rescue treatment of hypomobility during "off" episodes in clients with advanced PD

ALZHEIMER'S DISEASE

1. Which drugs listed for Alzheimer's disease are indicated for cognitive impairment?
2. Which drugs listed for Alzheimer's disease are indicated for neuropsychiatric symptoms (e.g., agitation, aggression, delusions, hallucinations)?
3. Which drugs should be reduced or discontinued in clients with renal impairment?
4. Cholinesterase inhibitors (e.g., donepezil) increase acetylcholine in the periphery and can cause anticholinergic side effects. What happens when acetylcholine is increased in the heart? What symptoms would the nurse expect to observe?
5. Drugs that block cholinergic receptors will reduce responses to cholinesterase inhibitors. What are examples of some of these drugs?
6. Memantine is in a separate drug class. What is its mechanism of action?

Tips for answering exam questions related to these medications (Rosenjack Burchum et al., 2016)

- The elevation of acetylcholine elicited by cholinesterase inhibitors (e.g., donepezil) of medications can cause serve cardiac symptoms such as severe bradycardia (with fainting spells, fall-related injuries, and the possibility of pacemaker placement)
- Memantine is approved only for moderate to severe AD and has no significant adverse effects

- There is no solid research evidence supporting that drugs, nutrients, supplements, exercise, cognitive training or other interventions can prevent AD or delay cognitive decline (p. 198).

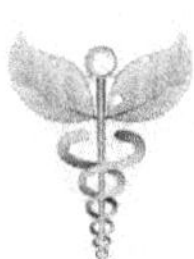

Integrative Therapy Caution

Herbal Medication: Ginkgo Biloba

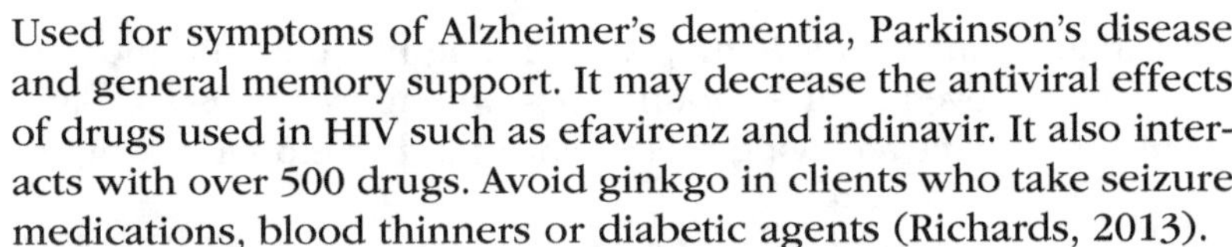

Used for symptoms of Alzheimer's dementia, Parkinson's disease and general memory support. It may decrease the antiviral effects of drugs used in HIV such as efavirenz and indinavir. It also interacts with over 500 drugs. Avoid ginkgo in clients who take seizure medications, blood thinners or diabetic agents (Richards, 2013).

MULTIPLE SCLEROSIS

1. Why should the nurse obtain baseline liver function tests and a complete blood count prior to the administration of interferon beta?
2. Which route is used for interferon beta formulations?
3. How often should the following interferon beta formulations be administered?
   i. Avonex
   ii. Rebif
   iii. Betaseron and Extavia
4. Flu-like reactions are common when interferon preparations are administered. What should the nurse recommend to reduce these symptoms?
5. SC administration can cause injection-site reactions. What would the nurse assess for in regards to a sc injection site reaction?
6. Outline how the nurse would assess for hepatotoxicity and myelosuppression often associated with interferon beta.
7. Dimethyl fumarate can increase risk of infection; therefore, it cannot be administered during an active infection. What should the nurse teach the client taking this medication in regards to recognizing infections? Can clients have live virus vaccines while taking this medication?
8. Flushing is associated with dimethyl fumarate, which medication can be administered 30 minutes prior to administration of this medication to prevent this side effect?
9. Glatiramer acetate causes uncomfortable and disturbing symptoms after the first 15-20 minutes of injection. What are these symptoms?
10. What is progressive multifocal leukoencephalopathy? Which drug is it associated with? What are the symptoms?
11. Natalizumab can harm the liver and cause hepatotoxicity. What are signs of hepatoxicity?

12. Fingolimod can cause severe bradycardia, especially after the first dose. If treatment is discontinued for two weeks or longer and restarted they should also be monitored again. How long should a client be observed by a health care provider after the first dose or after a disruption in treatment (where the drug is restarted again)? If a client develops bradycardia which drugs can be used to treat it? Based on this side effect, which cardiac medications should be avoided when clients are receiving this medication?
13. Fingolimod can cause macular edema. What are signs and symptoms of this condition?
14. Fingolimod can also cause liver injury, reduce lung function and increases the risk of infection (even after 2 months of stopping treatment). Create a teaching plan for a client receiving this medication to help with symptom recognition.
15. Can fingolimod be given to pregnant or breast-feeding women?
16. What would be signs of fingolimod toxicity?
17. Mitoxantrone can cause cardiac toxicity. What would be signs of this adverse effect?
18. Mitoxantrone can also cause urine and tissue discolouration. What colour does the urine, skin and sclera turn?

Tips for answering exam questions related to these medications (Rosenjack Burchum et al., 2016)

- Infection, hepatoxicity, myelosuppression are common side effects of these medications. Look for these indications in the question stem and potential answers.
- Focus in on harmful or drug-specific side effects when studying
- Life threatening adverse effects (e.g., Bradycardia associated with fingolimod) should be reviewed and treatment covered
- Fingolimod has very adverse side effects: bradycardia, macular edema, liver injury, effects on pregnancy and fetus, etc.—study the symptoms of these conditions and review associated lab results

DRUGS FOR EPILEPSY

1. Why should phenytoin NOT be administered faster than 50mg/min in adults?
2. What is the only IV fluid compatible with phenytoin?
3. What happens if extravasation occurs during a phenytoin infusion?
4. What is gingival hyperplasia and why does it occur with phenytoin administration? What medication can be given alongside phenytoin to help prevent this condition?
5. Phenytoin is a teratogen. What does this mean? What effects can it cause?
6. Phenytoin has several drug-to-drug interactions. Identify drugs that phenytoin will decrease therapeutic levels of and drugs that will increase plasma levels of phenytoin.
7. What are signs of phenytoin toxicity?

8. What happens if phenytoin is abruptly withdrawn?
9. What is purple glove syndrome associated with IV phenytoin administration?
10. Why should opioids, barbiturates and antihistamines be avoided in clients taking phenytoin therapy?
11. Phenytoin can cause a morbilliform (measles-like) rash that can lead to serious conditions such as Stevens-Johnson syndrome or toxic epidermal necrolysis. What should the nurse do in this situation?
12. What are potential hematologic effects associated with carbamazepine administration. Provide examples of signs and symptoms related to leukopenia, anemia, thrombocytopenia, aplastic anemia.
13. Valporic acid can cause life-threatening pancreatitis. What are signs of this condition?
14. Which drug does valporic acid raise the levels of? (*Hint, it is another drug used for epilepsy*)

Tips for answering exam questions related to these medications (Rosenjack Burchum et al., 2016)

- Severe dermatologic reactions can occur with these medications. Look for any indications that the client has a measles-like rash because it can advance to more serious conditions. Inform the health care provider immediately.
- These medications are commonly harmful during pregnancy and cause fetal defects. It is recommended that birth control is used and folic acid is taken in case of pregnancy (due to neural tube defects these medications cause).
- Other CNS depressants should be avoided (alcohol, opioids, benzodiazapines)
- Cessation of treatment frequently results in withdrawal seizures

---

Integrative Therapy Caution

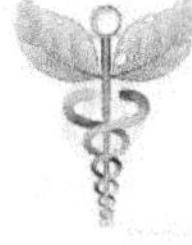

Herbal Medication: Evening Primrose Oil

May slow blood clotting and increase incidences of bleeding. This herb reacts with anti-seizure medications or phenothiazine drugs (Richards, 2013).

DRUGS FOR MUSCLE SPASM AND SPASTICITY

1. Make drug cards for Baclofen, Dantrolene and Diazepam
2. What can abrupt withdrawal of oral Baclofen result in?
3. What can abrupt withdrawal of intrathecal baclofen result in?
4. Identify signs of CNS depression that may be associated with this type of drug therapy.

Tips for answering exam questions related to these medications (Rosenjack Burchum et al., 2016)

- CNS depression associated with other medications is the most common and serious adverse effect of these medications
- Hepatic toxicity can also occur with the administration of dantrolene
- Rhabdomyolysis can occur when intrathecal baclofen is discontinued. Watch for signs such as increased myoglobin, paired with increased creatinine and BUN. Research treatment of rhabdomyolysis

PRACTICE QUESTIONS

Question 1

A client is being treated for poisoning from excessive doses of IV atropine. Which of the following Health Care Provider's orders should the nurse expect in this situation?

1. Neostigmine bromide 15 mg po once only
2. Physostigmine 2mg IM once only
3. Epinephrine 1mg IV direct once only
4. Metoprolol 25 mg po once only

Question 2

A client with Parkinson's Disease has been started on pramipexole 0.125 mg tid with meals. When teaching the client regarding this medication's adverse events what should the nurse include? **(Select all that apply)**

1. That sleep attacks characterized by overwhelming sleepiness may come without warning
2. To recognize signs and symptoms of agranulocytosis
3. The drug increases the risk of impulse control disorders
4. Combination with levodopa can cause orthostatic hypotension
5. To take the medication on an empty stomach

Question 3

A client taking Levodopa/Carbidopa has developed a tremor, twitching and dystonic movements. What is a nursing priority in this situation?

1. Stop the medication and notify the health care provider
2. Reduce the medication dose
3. Assess the client's airway and breathing
4. Ensure the client has a stable blood pressure

Question 4

A client is receiving valporic acid to control seizure activity. Which following clinical signs should the nurse observe for when administering this medication?

1. Cardiac dysrhythmias
2. Abdominal pain, nausea and elevated serum lipase levels
3. Potassium loses through excessive voiding
4. Signs of increased sedation

Question 5

A client with Multiple Sclerosis is receiving the first dose of fingolimod in an outpatient care clinic. What is a priority nursing intervention when administering the first dose of this medication?

1. To observe the client in the outpatient care clinic for at least 6 hours after the first dose because bradycardia may occur
2. Instruct the client that they are not to receive any live virus vaccines
3. To assess for progressive weakness on one side of the body
4. To observe for any excessive flushing of the skin or urticaria

Question 6

A client with severe Alzheimer's Disease takes memantine 10mg po bid with the assistance of his wife. The client's wife is concerned because her husband has been having bradycardic episodes and fainting. She asks the nurse to discontinue his memantine because of this. Which of the following statements by the nurse BEST demonstrates information regarding the adverse effects of memantine?

1. "Memantine has no adverse or life-threatening side effects, perhaps we should explore his other medications"
2. "Orthohypostatic hypotension is common with this medication"
3. "Bradycardia and syncope are indications that the dose of the medication is too high"
4. "Memantine depletes potassium reserves in the body this may be causing his cardiac symptoms"

Answers: Question 1: 2; Question 2: 1,3,4; Question 3: 1, Question 4: 2, Question 5: 1, Question 6: 1

Study Strategy

This study guide differs from other resources because formal rationale is not provided for the answers. **You need to determine the appropriate rationale for the correct answers by accessing the information in the question that may have inhibited your ability to answer the question correctly.** It is helpful to ask the following questions:

- What is the question asking? What are key words in the question query?
- What information do I need to know to answer this question correctly?
- How did I select my answer?
- Why were the other answers incorrect?
- Was I missing a piece of content knowledge that inhibited how I answered the question? If so, what should I target in on and study?

Additional Strategies for Working with the Pharmacology Study Guide Modules

Content review is essential for being successful at answering NCLEX-RN® exam questions focusing on pharmacology. The following tips will help you to navigate the breath of this content and to organize your study notes. **Remember that you need to do the work of solid content review in order to be successful in understanding pharmacological concepts. Do not rely on practice questions to teach you what you need to know regarding medications for the NCLEX-RN®- practice questions are a tool for consolidating knowledge not a primary way to study.**

1. Complete the exercises in this study guide and make notes. This guide has been designed to direct you to important content for medication review. When creating the study guide using my pharmacology textbook I used an educator's lens to pull out the most important information in order ensure client safety with drug administration. For example, when review differing drugs I focused on critical information and essential education for each drug. The review questions are designed to bring this information forward.
2. Find ways to colour code or organize medications according to the bodily system or pathology they are used for. This will help you with recalling information. This guide uses a systems approach to help you organize the vast amount of pharmacological review in a way that will help you understand key concepts and pathologies.
3. Create case studies or unique ways to remember classes of medications. It is always wise to study pharmacology in the context of pathology. Use case studies specifically for content that is new to you or more difficult. Case studies should be memorable, contain client information that is easy to remember, focus on adverse effects of medications and key aspects of client education.
4. It is helpful to find patterns in names in drugs- such as suffixes that are common. Highlight the endings of common terms and find strategies to remember the main side effects of these classes of medications.
5. Client teaching is essential in medication administration. Ensure that you review your client education chapter in your Fundamentals of Nursing textbook (e.g. Potter and Perry). You need to remember that the use of basic teaching and learning principles paired with your knowledge of medications can help you to better exam questions.
6. When you use practice questions find consistent strategies for reviewing questions that you get incorrect. For example, the summary drug tables presented in each module of this guide provide a structure for organizing information. Create a blank table with the drug classes named for each system. Write information or content that is tested in each drug class as you move through your practice resources. Highlight the medication names you

have seen in the practice questions on your summary table. Are there any patterns in the types of questions asked or the content tested? **Do be careful with this strategy- it is not a replacement for reviewing content.**

Conclusion

Strong pharmacological review will not only increase your chances of success on the NCLEX-RN® it will also strengthen your future nursing practice. The complexity of client care paired with the increase in co-morbidity and chronic disease management poses many challenges to pharmacological therapy. Nurses must be aware of potential drug-to-drug interactions, polypharmacy, and adverse events related to medications in order to keep their clients safe. I wish you all the best for your NCLEX-RN® exam and for your future nursing practice.

Best wishes,

Dr. Marnie Kramer-Kile

REFERENCES

Copstead, L.E & Banaski, J. (2013). *Pathophysiology* (5th ed). St. Louis: Elsevier.

Richards, J.S. (2013). Overview of herbal supplements. *Elite Continuing Education*, 46-72.

Rosenjack Burchum, J. & Rosenthal, L.D. (2016). *Lehne's pharmacology for nursing care* (9th edition). St. Louis: Elsevier.

Module 4

Drugs Affecting the Gastrointestinal System

TABLE OF CONTENTS

Introduction to the Transitioning to the NCLEX-RN® Pharmacology Guide: Drugs Affecting the Gastrointestinal (GI) System

The breadth and detail of the knowledge required of pharmacological concepts often overwhelms new graduates when they are beginning their exam preparation. The purpose of this pharmacology study guide is to help you work through the vast amount of pharmacological knowledge required for the NCLEX-RN® in a systematic and purposeful way. This guide organizes content using the current NCLEX-RN® Test Plan and provides specific strategies to address pharmacological areas of review which may challenge new graduates. **This is the fourth of twelve modules.** This is a working guide, so while key information will be presented and organized for review, it is up to you to do the detailed work of content review by answering the questions and exercises in each section. You can expect to see drugs described by their generic names on the exam. Due to the differences in drug trade names between the United States of America, Canada and other nations you should study drugs according to their generic names and develop strategies for remembering them.

This module is part of a comprehensive pharmacology study guide focusing on specific areas which may challenge NCLEX-RN® candidates. This includes drug-to-drug interactions, specific adverse reactions due to drug therapy and the potential reactions associated with herbal therapy and conventional medications. The content will be focused on a systems approach and will direct you towards important information within each drug class.

Structure of the Module

This module begins with an overview of the differing drug classes for the GI system. Additional areas for review that are specialized or affect multiple systems will also be highlighted:

1. Review questions and selected exercises will be constructed for each drug class to help pull out key concepts such as adverse events/side effects, specific client teaching and drug to drug interactions.
2. A summary chart of the drug classes in each system or theme will be provided for you to use alongside practice questions. As you move through practice questions, check off the specific medications you come across and if you require further review in each area. It is also helpful to make your own drug cards for specific medications. Keep the drug cards simple. Identify the drug class, the mechanism of action, two relevant (i.e., life threatening) or unique adverse effects that require monitoring and provide an outline for client teaching or specific nursing interventions for the medication.

Introduction to the Pharmacology Guide: Drugs Affecting the Gastrointestinal System

Structure of the Module

Advice for Studying Pharmacological Content for the NCLEX-RN®

Always start with areas you are NOT familiar with. For example, if you spent the majority of your time as a final practicum student/or nurse on a cardiology unit do not start in the Vascular and Cardiac Medications Module. It is common for students/graduates to move to areas of comfort when they are studying because it decreases their anxiety. However, your efforts should be targeted on what you don't know. Each Module in this guide has a summary table of drugs for each system. Highlight the drug classes that you are not familiar with and make it your priority to work through them. Do not spend time making drug cards for medications you already know. For example, most students are confident with furosemide administration and can critically think through concepts associated with the drug. Therefore, time does not need to be spent studying this medication. Only make drug cards for medications that are new to you. The review questions in this guide will direct you towards more detailed information of the medications that you are familiar with and focus on potential areas where exam questions may be asked.

This guide is set up using a **systems approach** for the following reasons: 1) most pharmacology textbooks use this approach to structure content so it will be easier to find the information you need to answer the review questions; 2) using a systems approach allows you to find commonalties in the side effects of drugs influencing a specific system, so you will see patterns arising as you work through this guide; and 3) a systems approach allows for the creation of overall drug summary tables, which will be included in each module of the guide and will provide you with a general sense of the medications you need to cover.

The following resources will aid you in answering questions posed in this guide. This includes:

1. **A pharmacology textbook.** This resource will contain more detailed information pertaining to drug classes and outline general nursing considerations for therapy. I have referenced a pharmacology textbook throughout the writing of this guide.
2. **A drug guide**. These are the guides commonly used for your clinical practice. These resources contain alphabetized drug information. Most importantly, they outline specific pharmacokinetic and pharmacodynamics properties of drugs. You will find information related to drug excretion, protein binding, and therapeutic index in these guides.
3. **An online drug repository** for more detailed information that may not be found in the two resources above. Sometimes it is difficult to find therapeutic index and protein binding for a drug. I have found the following website helpful for this: http://www.drugbank.ca/drugs

Module 4: Drugs Affecting the Gastrointestinal System

The most common drugs in this system focus on the treatment of **peptic ulcer disease**. Other focuses of treatment for the gastrointestinal system include **laxatives**, **anti-diarrheal** medications and **anti-emetics**. While the majority of these medications have limited side effects, they can potentiate issues with the absorption of medications. **It is helpful to think about these medications in regards to their indications, adverse events and client teaching**. These medications also have the potential for several different types of drug-to-drug interactions due to the fact that their mechanisms of action influence absorption in the GI system. Refer to Module 1: Understanding Drug-to-Drug Interactions to review how these medications influence the absorption of other medications.

Table 4.1: Summary of Drugs Affecting the Gastrointestinal System

DRUGS AFFECTING THE GASTROINTESTINAL SYSTEM		
Acid Controlling Agents **Antacids** 3 classes (magnesium, aluminium or calcium salts) • Use with caution or not at all in clients with renal failure. Magnesium may accumulate and cause toxicity. Excessive use can result in systemic alkalosis. Constipation is also a side effect. • Drug to drug interactions are common in this class of drugs **H2 Antagonists** (block 90% acid secretion) • Block glands in parietal cells in stomach which produce hydrogen ions and HCL. Compete with histamine for binding. • Cimetidine (can induce erectile dysfunction, gynecomastia), Famotidine, Nizatidine, Ranitidine • Adverse effects all drugs: depression, hallucinations, increased prolactin, jaundice, increased BUN, LFTs, creatinine, agranulocytosis, thrombocytopenia, neutropenia, aplastic anemia, exfoliative dermatitis	**Antidiarrheal** **Absorbents**—coat wall of GI tract, bind causative bacteria to the surface & eliminate it via the stool (*activated charcoal, aluminum hydroxide, bismuth subsalicylate*) • S/E: increased bleeding time, hearing loss, tinnitus, metallic taste, blue gum (all related to bismuth subsalicylate as it contains ASA) **Anticholinergic/Antispasmodics** • decrease peristalsis, slowing movement- used in combination with absorbents/opiates (*atropine, hyoscyamine, hyoscine)* • S/E: urinary retention, erectile dysfunction, hypotension, bradycardia, blurred vision, increased eye pressure **Intestinal Flora Modifiers** • create an unfavourable environment for overgrowth of harmful fungi & bacteria (lactobacillus acidophilus). Typically given for uncomplicated diarrhea. **Opiates** • decrease bowel motility, allowing water/electrolytes to absorb decreasing stool frequency and volume (*codeine, diphenoxylate, loperamide*) • S/E: sedation, respiratory depression, bradycardia, palpitations, hypotension, flushing, urticarial	**Laxatives** **Bulk forming**—absorbs water, increases bulk, distends bowel to initiate reflex bowel activity (*psyllium, polycarbophil, methylcellulose*) **Emollient**—stool softeners or lubricant laxatives (*docusate salts, mineral oils*) **Hyperosmotic** • increases fecal water content, results in distension, increased peristalsis, evacuation (*polyethylene glycol, lactulose, sorbitol, glycerin*) **Saline** • increases osmotic pressure in small intestine inhibits absorption and increasing water/electrolyte secretions, resulting in watery stool, promotes peristalsis/evacuation **Stimulant** • stimulates nerves in the intestines, resulting in increased peristalsis, increase fluid in colon, increases bulk & softens stool (*castor oil, senna, anthraquinones*)

<table>
<tr>
<td>Proton Pump Inhibitors (block all acid secretion)
• PPIs irreversibly bind to H+/K+ ATPase enzyme preventing movement of hydrogen ions out of parietal cells.
• Lansoprazole, omeprazole, rabeprazole, pantoprazole, esomeprazole (may be given to clients with h. pylori)

Sucralfate
• Binds directly to the surface of ulcers forming a protective barrier
• Safe drug—S/E: dry mouth, constipation, nausea</td>
<td></td>
<td></td>
</tr>
<tr>
<td>Antiemetics

Serotonin Receptor Antagonists (Ondansetron)
Glucocorticoids (methylprednisolone, dexamethasone)
Substance P/Neurokinin$_1$ Antagonists (Aprepitant)
Benzodiazepines (lorazepam)
Dopamine Antagonists (phenothiazines)
Cannabinoids (dronabinol, nabilone)
Anticholinergics (Scopolamine-motion sickness)
Antihistamines (Dimenhydrinate-motion sickness)</td>
<td>Drugs for Inflammatory Bowel Disease

5-Aminosalicylates (sulfasalazine, mesalamine, olsalazine, balsalazide)
Glucocorticoids
Immunosuppressants
• Thiopurines: Azathioprine & Mercaptopurine
• Cyclosporine
• Methotrexate
Immunomodulators
Infliximab (Remicade)</td>
<td>Prokinetic Agents

Metoclopramide (Reglan, Maxeran)
Cisapride (Propulsid)

Palifermin (first drug approved to decreasing oral mucositis due to chemoradiotherapy)</td>
</tr>
</table>

PEPTIC ULCER DISEASE

Peptic ulcers are caused by two primary mechanisms: 1) *H. pylori* infections and 2) Nonsteroidal Anti-inflammatory Drugs (NSAID) therapy. Common drug classes are listed below for the treatment of peptic ulcer disease and prototype drugs are posted. **It is helpful to start by mapping out the care of a client with Peptic Ulcer Disease before starting review on this section.**

- **Antibiotics:** amoxicillin/clarithromycin/omeprazole (used to make gastric pH more neutral so antibiotic therapy will work)
- **H2-Receptor Antagonists:** cimetidine
- **Proton Pump Inhibitors:** omeprazole
- **Mucosal Protectants:** sucralfate
- **Antacids:** aluminium hydroxide/magnesium hydroxide

REVIEW QUESTIONS

The following table highlights antibiotics employed for *H. pylori* infections. **Note that these medications are always given in a combination because none of them are effective in eradicating *H. pylori* alone—2-3 antibiotics are recommended** (Rosenjack Burchum et al., 2016, p. 951). Typically, a 10-day course is sufficient for eradication of *H. pylori* and is slightly better with a 14-day course. Complete the information in the table to gain a better understanding of the indications for these medications for the treatment of *H. pylori* infections:

Antibiotic	Action	Nursing Considerations
Clarithromycin (Biaxin)		
Amoxicillin		
Bismuth compounds		
Tetracycline		
Metronidazole (Flagyl)		
Tinidazole (Tindamax)		

*Typically a clarithromycin-based triple therapy consisting of: <u>clarithromycin</u> + <u>amoxicillin</u> + a <u>proton pump inhibitor</u> is the preferred treatment for the treatment of *H. pylori* infections.

H2-RECEPTOR ANTAGONISTS

Cimetidine (Tagmet) is used to suppress basal acid secretion and secretion stimulated by gastrin and acetylcholine. It is given IV, IM and orally. All routes reach comparable blood levels of the drug, but if it is taken orally with meals, absorption will be slowed and results prolonged (Rosenjack Burchum et al., 2016, p. 952).

1. What are the therapeutic uses of this drug?
2. Cimetidine crosses the blood-brain barrier (with some difficulty) but CNS side effects can occur. What are these potential side effects?
3. **One of the most important things to know about Cimetidine is that it inhibits hepatic drug-metabolizing enzymes and can cause other drug levels to rise.** There are four drugs that are of serious concern if they are administered with Cimetidine because they have narrow safety margins. Which drugs are these?
4. How far apart should the dosing of Cimetidine and antacids be spaced?
5. Ranitidine, famotidine and nizatidine have less drug-to-drug interactions than cimetidine. **Create drug cards for each of these medications.**

PROTON PUMP INHIBITORS (PPI)

Common drugs: *Omeprazole, Esomeprazole, Lansoprazole, Dexlansoprazole, Rabeprazole, Pantoprazole*

Although these drugs are generally well-tolerated, they can have severe drug-to-drug interactions.

Omeprazole: by elevating gastric pH, omeprazole can reduce the absorption of some important HIV/AIDS medications: atazanavir (Reyataz), delavirdine (Rescriptor) and nelfinavir (Viracept). Reducing gastric pH can decrease the absorption of ketoconazole and itraconazole (antifungal drugs).

a. What effects can omeprazole and other PPI's have on the drug Clopidogrel (Plavix)?
b. How does long-term therapy of lansoprazole and pantoprazole influence magnesium levels in the body?

OTHER ANTIULCER DRUGS

1. What is the mechanism of action of sucralfate? Is sucralfate actually absorbed into the blood stream?
2. Sucralfate can impede the absorption of some drugs, how can these interactions be minimized? Which drugs are of the most concern if their absorption is impeded?
3. Misoprostol is given for the prevention of gastric ulcers caused by long-term therapy with NSAIDS. It also has another use in the context of inducing

labour. What is this? Misoprostol can also be combined with another drug to induce a medical termination of pregnancy; which drug is this?

4. Based on these other potential uses, is misoprostol given to pregnant women?

ANTACIDS

There are four major classes of antacids: 1) Aluminum compounds, 2) magnesium compounds, 3) calcium compounds and 4) sodium compounds (Rosenjack Burchum et al., 2016).

1. What are common adverse effects of antacids?
2. What is sodium loading? Identify types of antacids that increase the risk of this complication.
3. Do antacids raise or drop gastric pH? How does this influence the absorption of other drugs and how long should you wait before giving other drugs after an antacid?
4. What is milk-alkali syndrome and which family of antacid drugs cause it?
5. Complete the following matching exercise:

Antacid	Treatment Indications/Side Effects
Aluminum hydroxide	May cause acid rebound or milk-alkali syndrome, releases CO2
Magnesium hydroxide	Not used routinely for ulcers; used to treat acidosis and to alkalinize urine; high risk of sodium loading; releases CO2
Calcium Carbonate	Can cause hypophosphatemia; can treat hyperphosphatemia
Sodium Bicarbonate	Can cause magnesium toxicity (CNS depression) in patients with renal impairment

Adapted from Rosenjack Burchum & Rosenthal (2016). Lehne's pharmacology for nursing care (9th ed.). St. Louis: Elsevier. p. 959. Answers: 1c, 2d, 3a, 4b

LAXATIVES

1. Complete the following review table for common laxatives:

Drug Class for Laxatives	Prototype Drug	Drug Action	Specific Teaching Interventions
Bulk-Forming	Methylcellulose		
Surfactants	Docusate sodium		
Stimulant Laxatives	Bisacodyl		
Osmotic Laxatives	Magnesium hydroxide		
Chloride Channel Activator	Lubiprostone		

2. What is lactulose and what are the indications for this drug therapy?
3. Identify laxatives used for bowel cleansing prior to colonoscopy.
4. Laxative abuse is common in many clients. What are signs of laxative abuse and what specific client teaching should be completed?

Tips for answering exam questions related to these medications (Rosenjack Burchum et al., 2016, p. 969-970)

- Osmotic laxatives can lead to water losses; assess for dehydration and teach client to increase fluid intake
- In clients with renal impairment, magnesium can accumulate to toxic levels with osmotic laxatives
- Sodium absorption with osmotic laxatives (sodium phosphate in particular) can cause fluid retention: if a client has heart failure, hypertension or edema these conditions may worsen—these disorders are contraindications to the administration of sodium phosphate
- Bulk forming laxatives should be administered with fluid to avoid esophageal obstruction
- Laxatives are contraindicated for individuals with: abdominal pain, nausea, cramps and other symptoms of appendicitis, regional enteritis, diverticulitis, and ulcerative colitis. They are also contraindicated for clients with surgical abdomen, fecal impaction and obstruction of the bowel.

ANTIEMETIC DRUGS

1. Complete the following table:

Drug Class and Prototype Drug	Mechanism of Action	Special Considerations/ Client Teaching
Serotonin Receptor Antagonists (ondansetron)		
Glucocorticoids (methylprednisolone, dexamethasone)		
Substance P/Neurokinin$_1$ Antagonists (aprepitant)		
Benzodiazapines (lorazepam)		

Dopamine Antagonists (phenothiazines)		
Cannabinoids (dronabinol, nabilone)		
Anticholingerics (scopolamine—motion sickness)		
Antihistamines (dimenhydrinate—motion sickness)		

2. Which drugs are recommended for the management of chemotherapy induced vomiting?
3. Which drugs are recommended for nausea and vomiting during pregnancy?
4. Which drugs are recommended for motion sickness?

Tips for answering exam questions related to these medications (Rosenjack Burchum et al., 2016):

- Droperidol and Ondansetron can cause QT prolongation, all clients undergoing this drug therapy should have a ECG completed for evaluation of underlying heart disease or prolonged QT (Droperidol is only approved in the US)
- Lorazepam is used for sedation, suppression of anticipatory emesis and production of anterograde amnesia
- Phenothiazines can cause extrapyramidal reactions, anticholinergic effects, hypotension and sedation. Lorazepam can be given as an adjunct to this therapy to control extrapyramidal reactions caused by these drugs.
- Promethazine (Phenothaizine drug class) is the most widely used antiemetic in young children, despite its adverse side effects of respiratory depression and local tissue injury and despite the availability of safer alternatives; it is not to be given to children under the age of 2, and subcutaneous administration is contraindicated
- Aprepitant can decrease levels of ethinyl estradiol found in oral contraceptives—another form of birth control should be used if client is taking both of these medications
- Aprepitant can also decrease warfarin levels—this is to be taken into account in clients receiving warfarin therapy

- Ondansetron is more effective when combined with dexamethasone
- Methylprednisolone and dexamethasone are used for their antiemetic properties but are not approved by the FDA for this use—both drugs are administered IV in this context

ANTIDIARRHEAL AGENTS

Management of diarrhea is focused on: 1) diagnosis and treatment of the underlying disease, 2) replacement of lost water or salts, 3) relief of cramping and 4) reducing passage of unformed stools (p. 977). Therefore, antidiarrheal drugs focus on the treatment of diarrhea itself and the treatment of the underlying cause of the condition.

1. Identify common opioid antidiarrheal agents. It is important to note the dose for these medications. What are expected side effects of these drugs?
2. Loperamide is a commonly used antidiarrheal agent, which type of opioid is it related to? Why can't it be bought over-the-counter?
3. Which bacteria is primarily responsible for traveler's diarrhea?
4. Should antidiarrheal agents be given to clients with a known clostridium difficile-associated infection in the bowel?

DRUGS GIVEN FOR INFLAMMATORY BOWEL DISEASE

1. 5-Aminosalicylates are used to treat mild to moderate ulcerative colitis and Crohn's disease and to maintain remission after symptoms have subsided. Drugs available include: sulfasalazine, olsalazine, mesalamine, and balsalazide. What are potential adverse effects related to sulfasalazine? Why should complete blood counts be ordered for clients on this therapy?
2. What are consequences of long-term glucocorticoid therapy? How does oral budesonide (Entocort) work to treat Crohn's disease?
3. What are the most common adverse effects associated with Cyclosporine? (*remember cyclosporine is also used to prevent organ rejection in allogenic transplant*)
4. Cyclosporine has several drug-to-drug interactions that can either accelerate its metabolism (causing levels to fall) or raise cyclosporine levels, resulting in toxicity. Which drugs may increase the chance of toxicity with cyclosporine?
5. Lower doses of methotrexate can be used to treat Crohn's disease to promote short-term remission and thereby reduce the need for glucocorticoid therapy (p. 982). What are nursing considerations for a client receiving methotrexate?
6. Immunomodulators such as infliximab (Remicade), certolizumab and adalimumab are generally considered second-line agents for the treatment of inflammatory bowel disease; some health care providers, however, are using them early in treatment. What are serious side effects of infliximab (Remicade)? What disease can infliximab increase the risk of?

Tips for answering exam questions related to these medications (Rosenjack Burchum et al., 2016):

- Glucocorticoids are indicated for induction of remission, not long term maintenance
- Immunosuppressants are generally reserved for clients who have not responded to traditional therapy—they can take up to 6 months to work

PROKINETIC AGENTS

1. What are the two actions of metoclopramide (Reglan, Maxeran)? Which extrapyramidal side effect can be caused by long-term use of metoclopramide? What are the symptoms of this condition? Why is this drug NOT given in cases of GI obstruction, perforation or hemorrhage?
2. Cisapride (Propulsid) is a drug that was voluntarily taken off the US market in July 2000 due to its association with fatal cardiac dysrhythmias. It is available today but considered a drug of last resort. Which specific assessments would a client need to undergo prior to being started on this medication?
3. Palifermin (Kepivance) is the first drug to be approved for treating oral mucositis (a complication of chemotherapy). What is its mechanism of action? (*note it is only indicated for clients with hematologic malignancies, those receiving high-dose chemotherapy and whole-body irradiation*; p. 984).

PRACTICE QUESTIONS

Question 1

A client receiving chemotherapy has been prescribed ondansetron to treat nausea and vomiting. The client has become critically ill and is in the intensive care unit for low electrolyte levels. What is a priority nursing intervention for this client while they remain on this medication?

1. To discontinue the medication while in the intensive care unit
2. To assess for potential extrapyramidal effects
3. To ensure cardiac monitoring for QT prolongation
4. To assess for anticholinergic side effects

Question 2

A female client diagnosed with Ulcerative Colitis is started on sulfasalazine 500mg delayed-release oral tablets once daily. What is a priority nursing intervention when caring for clients taking this medication?

1. Diarrhea is common and should be treated with increased fluid intake
2. Ensure that a CBC is obtained periodically while on medication therapy
3. Teach the client that they cannot become pregnant while taking the medication
4. QT prolongation can occur

Question 3

A female client has been prescribed misoprostol to prevent gastric ulcers caused by long-term therapy of the NSAIDs she is taking for rheumatoid arthritis. What is a critical factor that the nurse must assess for prior to starting this medication?

1. History of QT prolongation or episodes of syncope
2. Negative serum pregnancy test results within 2 weeks before beginning therapy
3. Assess electrolyte levels prior to administration
4. Presence of existing constipation or abdominal pain

Question 4

A client has been started on pantoprazole for peptic ulcer disease. The client is confused as to when to take the medication during the day. What should the nurse recommend?

1. To take pantoprazole just before eating
2. To take pantoprazole after eating
3. To always take pantoprazole on an empty stomach
4. Pantoprazole may be taken without regard to food

Question 5
A client is taking a bulk-forming laxative to treat constipation. What should the nurse recommend for clients taking this medication?

1. This medication can cause discolouration of the urine to take yellowish-brown or pink
2. This medication is a powerful laxative and should not be used to treat routine constipation
3. This medication should be taken within 1 hour after ingesting milk or antacids
4. To take the medication with a full glass of water to prevent esophageal obstruction

Question 6
A male client has been started on cimetidine for the treatment of a gastric ulcer. Which of the following side effects is the client at risk for while taking this medication? **Select all that Apply.**

1. Gynecomastia
2. Rebound acid secretion
3. Risk of osteoporosis
4. Reduced libido
5. Impotence

Answers: Question 1(3), Question 2(2), Question 3 (2), Question 4(4), Question 5(4), Question 6 (1,4,5)

Study Strategy

This study guide differs from other resources because formal rationale is not provided for the answers. **You need to determine the appropriate rationale for the correct answers by accessing the information in the question that may have inhibited your ability to answer the question correctly.** It is helpful to ask the following questions:

- What is the question asking? What are key words in the question query?
- What information do I need to know to answer this question correctly?
- How did I select my answer?
- Why were the other answers incorrect?
- Was I missing a piece of content knowledge that inhibited how I answered the question? If so, what should I target in on and study?

Additional Strategies for Working with the Pharmacology Study Guide Modules

Content review is essential for being successful at answering NCLEX-RN® exam questions focusing on pharmacology. The following tips will help you to navigate the breath of this content and to organize your study notes. **Remember that you need to do the work of solid content review in order to be successful in understanding pharmacological concepts. Do not rely on practice questions to teach you what you need to know regarding medications for the**

NCLEX-RN®- practice questions are a tool for consolidating knowledge not a primary way to study.

1. Complete the exercises in this study guide and make notes. This guide has been designed to direct you to important content for medication review. When creating the study guide I used an educator's lens to pull out the most important information in order ensure client safety with drug administration. For example, when review differing drugs I focused on critical information and essential education for each drug. The review questions are designed to bring this information forward.
2. Find ways to colour code or organize medications according to the bodily system or pathology they are used for. This will help you with recalling information. This guide uses a systems approach to help you organize the vast amount of pharmacological review in a way that will help you understand key concepts and pathologies.
3. Create case studies or unique ways to remember classes of medications. It is always wise to study pharmacology in the context of pathology. Use case studies specifically for content that is new to you or more difficult. Case studies should be memorable, contain client information that is easy to remember, focus on adverse effects of medications and key aspects of client education.
4. It is helpful to find patterns in names in drugs- such as suffixes that are common. Highlight the endings of common terms and find strategies to remember the main side effects of these classes of medications.
5. Client teaching is essential in medication administration. Ensure that you review your client education chapter in your Fundamentals of Nursing textbook (e.g. Potter and Perry). You need to remember that the use of basic teaching and learning principles paired with your knowledge of medications can help you to better exam questions.
6. When you use practice questions find consistent strategies for reviewing questions that you get incorrect. For example, the summary drug tables presented in each module of this guide provide a structure for organizing information. Create a blank table with the drug classes named for each system. Write information or content that is tested in each drug class as you move through your practice resources. Highlight the medication names you have seen in the practice questions on your summary table. Are there any patterns in the types of questions asked or the content tested? **Do be careful with this strategy- it is not a replacement for reviewing content.**

Conclusion

Strong pharmacological review will not only increase your chances of success on the NCLEX-RN® it will also strengthen your future nursing practice. The complexity of client care paired with the increase in co-morbidity and chronic disease management poses many challenges to pharmacological therapy. Nurses must be aware of potential drug-to-drug interactions, polypharmacy, and adverse events related to medications in order to keep their clients safe. I wish you all the best for your NCLEX-RN® exam and for your future nursing practice.

Best wishes,

Dr. Marnie Kramer-Kile

REFERENCES

Copstead, L.E & Banaski, J. (2013). *Pathophysiology* (5th ed). St. Louis: Elsevier.

Richards, J.S. (2013). Overview of herbal supplements. *Elite Continuing Education*, 46-72.

Rosenjack Burchum, J. & Rosenthal, L.D. (2016). *Lehne's pharmacology for nursing care* (9th edition). St. Louis: Elsevier.

Module 5

Vascular and Cardiac Medications

TABLE OF CONTENTS

Tables and Figures

TABLE OF CONTENTS

Tables and Figures

Introduction to the Transitioning to the NCLEX-RN® Pharmacology Guide: Vascular and Cardiac Medications

The breadth and detail of the knowledge required of pharmacological concepts often overwhelms new graduates when they are beginning their exam preparation. The purpose of this pharmacology study guide is to help you work through the vast amount of pharmacological knowledge required for the NCLEX-RN® in a systematic and purposeful way. This guide organizes content using the current NCLEX-RN® Test Plan and provides specific strategies to address pharmacological areas of review which may challenge new graduates. **This is the fifth of twelve modules.** This is a working guide, so while key information will be presented and organized for review, it is up to you to do the detailed work of content review by answering the questions and exercises in each section. You can expect to see drugs described by their generic names on the exam. Due to the differences in drug trade names between the United States of America, Canada and other countries you should study drugs according to their generic names and develop strategies for remembering them.

This module is part of a comprehensive pharmacology study guide focusing on specific areas which may challenge NCLEX-RN® candidates. This includes drug-to-drug interactions, specific adverse reactions due to drug therapy and the potential reactions associated with herbal therapy and conventional medications. The content will be focused on a systems approach and will direct you towards important information within each drug class.

Structure of the Module

This module begins with an overview of the differing drug classes for the cardiac and vascular system. Additional areas for review that are specialized or affect multiple systems will also be highlighted:

1. Review questions and selected exercises will be constructed for each drug class to help pull out key concepts such as adverse events/side effects, specific client teaching and drug to drug interactions.
2. A summary chart of the drug classes in each system or theme will be provided for you to use alongside practice questions. As you move through practice questions, check off the specific medications you come across and if you require further review in each area. It is also helpful to make your own drug cards for specific medications. Keep the drug cards simple. Identify the drug class, the mechanism of action, two relevant (i.e., life threatening) or unique adverse effects that require monitoring and provide an outline for client teaching or specific nursing interventions for the medication.

Advice for Studying Pharmacological Content for the NCLEX-RN®

Always start with areas you are NOT familiar with. For example, if you spent the majority of your time as a final practicum student on a respiratory unit do not start in the Drugs Affecting the Respiratory System Module. It is common for students/graduates to move to areas of comfort when they are studying because it decreases their anxiety. However, your efforts should be targeted on what you don't know. Each Module in this guide has a summary table of drugs for each system. Highlight the drug classes that you are not familiar with and make it your priority to work through them. Do not spend time making drug cards for medications you already know. For example, most students are confident with furosemide administration and can critically think through concepts associated with the drug. Therefore, time does not need to be spent studying this medication. Only make drug cards for medications that are new to you. The review questions in this guide will direct you towards more detailed information of the medications that you are familiar with and focus on potential areas where exam questions may be asked.

This guide is set up using a **systems approach** for the following reasons: 1) most pharmacology textbooks use this approach to structure content so it will be easier to find the information you need to answer the review questions; 2) using a systems approach allows you to find commonalties in the side effects of drugs influencing a specific system, so you will see patterns arising as you work through this guide; and 3) a systems approach allows for the creation of overall drug summary tables, which will be included in each module of the guide and will provide you with a general sense of the medications you need to cover.

The following resources will aid you in answering questions posed in this guide. This includes:

1. **A pharmacology textbook.** This resource will contain more detailed information pertaining to drug classes and outline general nursing considerations for therapy. I have referenced a pharmacology textbook throughout the writing of this guide.
2. **A drug guide**. These are the guides commonly used for your clinical practice. These resources contain alphabetized drug information. Most importantly, they outline specific pharmacokinetic and pharmacodynamics properties of drugs. You will find information related to drug excretion, protein binding, and therapeutic index in these guides.
3. **An online drug repository** for more detailed information that may not be found in the two resources above. Sometimes it is difficult to find therapeutic index and protein binding for a drug. I have found the following website helpful for this: http://www.drugbank.ca/drugs

Module 5: Vascular and Cardiac Medications

This Module focuses on medications given for hypertension and common cardiac conditions. There are two drug tables listed and some of the drugs overlap. However, it is important to remember why the medication is being used and how it influences the pathology it is prescribed for.

Table 5.1: Drugs for the Treatment of Hypertension

Beta Blockers Acebutolol Atenolol Betazolol Bisoprolol Metoprolol Nadolol Nebivolol Penbutolol Pindolol Propranolol Timolol	**Alpha$_1$ Blockers** Doxazosin Prazosin Terazosin **Alpha/Beta Blockers** Carvedilol Labetalol **Centrally Acting Alpha$_2$ Agonists** Clonidine Guanabenz Guanfacine Methyldopa	**Adrenergic Neuron Blockers** Reserpine **ACE Inhibitors** Benazepril Captopril Enalapril Fosinopril Lisinopril Moexipril Perindopril Quinapril Ramipril Trandolapril
Angiotension II Receptor Blockers Azilsartan Candesartan Eprosartan Irbesartan Losartan Olmesartan Telmisartan Valsartan	**Direct Renin Inhibitor** Aliskiren **Aldosterone Antagonists** Eplerenone Spironolactone **Direct-Acting Vasodilators** Hydralazine Minoxidil	**Calcium Channel Blockers** Amlodipine Diltiazem Felodipine Isradipine Nicardipine Nifedipine

REVIEW QUESTIONS

The first set of review questions will focus on drug classes directly related to the treatment of hypertension. Other drug classes that have other indications for cardiac disease will be covered in the next section. Please note that diuretics are used to treat hypertension. Questions specific to these medications are included in the Renal Medication Module of this guide.

In order to better understand the mechanism of action of medications used to treat hypertension it is helpful to review the sites of drug action and the effects produced. This is outlined in the table below:

Table 5.2 Mechanisms of Action of Antihypertensive Medications

Site of Action	Effect of Antihypertensive Medications
Brainstem	Antihypertensive medications may act on the brainstem to reduce sympathetic outflow. This results in vasodilation, decreased myocardial contractility, and decreased heart rate. Dilation of arterioles reduces vascular resistance, while dilation of the veins reduces BP by decreasing venous return to the heart.
Sympathetic Ganglia	Blockade of ganglia reduces sympathetic stimulation of heart and blood vessels. Medications that produce ganglionic effects are very potent and rarely used. The last available drug mecamylamine was voluntarily removed from the market in 2009.
Terminals of Adrenergic Nerves	Antihypertensive medications may work at the adrenergic nerve terminals decreasing the release of norepinephrine. This results in decreased sympathetic stimulation of heart and blood vessels. These drug are known as adrenergic neuron blocking agents—reserpine is the only drug in this class still on the market.
Beta1 Adrenergic Receptors on the Heart	Blocking beta1 prevents sympathetic stimulation of the heart. decreasing heart rate and myocardial contractility.
Alpha1 Adrenergic Receptors on Blood Vessels	Blocking alpha1 receptors promotes dilation of arterioles (decreasing peripheral resistance) and veins (reducing preload).
Vascular Smooth Muscle	Antihypertensive drugs may also act directly on vascular smooth muscle to cause relaxation- sodium nitroprusside is used for hypertensive emergencies, while the other drugs in this class are for chronic hypertension.
Renal Tubules	Diuretics act on renal tubules to promote salt and water excretion, thereby decreasing blood volume and BP falls

Adapted from: Rosenjack Burchum, J. & Rosenthal, L.D. (2016). Lehne's pharmacology for nursing care (9th edition). St. Louis: Elsevier, p. 503.

Drugs for Treatment of Hypertension

ALPHA$_1$ BLOCKERS

1. Create drug cards for the two common medications in this drug class: doxazosin and terazosin.

2. Orthostatic hypotension is a primary concern with these medications, particularly with the first dose. How should the nurse assess for this side effect?
3. It is recommended that, in order to counteract the orthostatic hypotension associated with these medications, the first dose should be given at bedtime. What is the rationale for this intervention?
4. Both doxazosin and terazosin cause orthostatic hypotension, reflex tachycardia and nasal congestion. Terazosin has one other prominent side effect, what is it?

ALPHA/BETA BLOCKERS

1. Carvedilol and labetalol block both alpha and beta receptors. How does this contribute to the management of hypertension?
2. Both are considered nonselective beta blockers as well. What conditions can these types of medications precipitate?
3. Create drug cards for both of these medications.

CENTRALLY ACTING ALPHA$_2$ AGONISTS

1. Which side effect occurs when clonidine is abruptly discontinued?
2. What are adverse effects associated with methyldopa?
3. In cases of hemolytic anemia associated with methyldopa, which lab test must also be positive?

ADRENERGIC NEURON BLOCKERS

1. Reserpine is the only drug in this class still available. What are the mechanism of action of this medication?
2. Reserpine depletes serotonin and catecholamines from neurons in the central nervous system. What condition results from this?
3. Why would this medication be contraindicated in individuals with clients with a history of depressive illness?

DIRECT-ACTING VASODILATORS

1. These medications act directly on arterioles and NOT veins. Why would this decrease the risk of orthostatic hypotension?
2. Hydralazine can cause a syndrome resembling systemic lupus erythematosus (SLE). What would be signs of this side effect of this drug?
3. Minoxidil can cause fluid retention potentially leading to pericardial effusion. What would be symptoms of this side effect?
4. Minoxidil also causes another rare and unique side effect. What is it?

DIRECT RENIN INHIBITORS

1. Only one DRI drug is available on the market, aliskiren. Why is this medication contraindicated in clients with type 2 diabetes mellitus who are also receiving ACE Inhibitors?

ALDOSTERONE ANTAGONISTS

1. How does this class of medications act to decrease hypertension?
2. Only two agents are available in this drug class: eplerenone and spironolactone. Which electrolyte do these medications INCREASE in the body?

Table 5.3 Drugs for the Treatment of Various Cardiac Disorders

Beta Blockers (MI, HF, Class II Antidysrhythmics) Acebutolol Atenolol Betazolol Bisoprolol Metoprolol Nadolol Nebivolol Penbutolol Pindolol Propranolol Timolol	**Calcium Channel Blockers (HTN, Vasospasm, Class IV Antidysrhythmics)** Amlodipine Diltiazem Felodipine Isradipine Nicardipine Nifedipine Ranolazine (anti-anginal medication) **Cardiac Glycosides** Digoxin	**Antidysrhythmic Drugs** **Class 1A** Quinidine Procainamide Disopyramide **Class 1B** lIdocaine Phenytoin Mexiletine **Class 1C** Flecainide Propafenone
ACE Inhibitors Benazepril Captopril Enalapril Fosinopril Lisinopril Moexipril Perindopril Quinapril Ramipril Trandolapril	**Angiotension II Receptor Blockers** Azilsartan Candesartan Eprosartan Irbesartan Losartan Olmesartan Telmisartan Valsartan	**Class III: Potassium Channel Blockers** Amiodarone Dronedarone Sotalol Dofetilide Ibutilide **Other Antidysrhythmic Drugs** Adenosine Digoxin
Nitrates Nitroglycern Isosorbide Mononitrate Isosorbide Dinitrate	**Antiplatelets** Aspirin Clopidogrel Prasugrel Ticagrelor Ticlopidine	**Anticoagulants** Heparin (unfractionated) Low- molecular weight heparins Enoxaparin (sc) Dalteparin (sc) Fondaparinux (sc) Warfarin (po)

HMG-CoA Reductase Inhibitors Lovastatin Atorvastatin Fluvastation Pitavastatin Pravastatin Rosuvastatin Simvastatin **Bile-Acid Sequestrants** Colesevelam **Others** Nicotinic acid Ezetimibe	**Glycoprotein IIb/IIIa Receptor Antagonists** Abeiximab Eptifibatide Tirofiban **Other Antiplatelet Drugs** Dipyridamole Cilostazol **Thrombolytic Drugs** Alteplase Reteplase Tenecteplase	**Direct Thrombin Inhibitors** Dabigatran Etexilate (po) Argatroban (IV) Bivalirudin (IV) Desirudin (sc) **Direct Factor Xa Inhibitors** Rivaroxaban (po) Apixaban (po) **Antithrombin (AT)** Recombinant human AT (IV) Plasma derived AT (IV) **Antiplatelet** Aspirin

The remainder of the review questions will focus on the drug classes identified in the table above. Remember that these drugs have varying indications for the treatment of cardiac disease, hypertension, dysrhythmias, angina, etc. To help you to conceptualize the uses of each of the medication classes listed in Table 5.3 a summary table of common drug classes for the treatment of angina, myocardial infarction, heart failure and dysrhythmias will be provided (Table 5.4). The review questions below will focus on general indications and nursing interventions for each drug class. The questions will also cue you to review some of the more pertinent adverse effects, drug-to-drug interactions and specific client teaching for some of the medications in each class.

REVIEW QUESTIONS

Drugs for Common Cardiac Conditions and Hypertension

CALCIUM CHANNEL BLOCKERS

The role of calcium in vascular smooth muscle is to contract smooth muscle, calcium channels are blocked in order to elicit vasodilation. At therapeutic doses CCB act selectively on peripheral arterioles, arteries and arterioles of the heart, they have no significant effect on veins (p. 485). CCB through their mechanism of action decrease the contractile force of the heart, reduce heart rate and decrease velocity of conduction through the AV node. In the heart calcium channels are coupled to $beta_1$-adrenergic receptors, when cardiac $beta_1$ receptors are activated, calcium influx is enhanced—therefore, when $beta_1$ receptors are blocked calcium influx is suppressed. There are two classifications of CCB: 1) agents that act on vascular smooth muscle and the heart, and 2) agents that act mainly on vascular smooth muscle.

Agents that Act On Vascular Smooth Muscle and the Heart

Verapamil and Diltiazem

1. What are the 5 direct effects of verapamil on the heart and blood vessels?
2. What are the therapeutic uses of verapamil?
3. Verapamil is generally well-tolerated in clients with healthy hearts, however, in clients with certain cardiac diseases verapamil can exacerbate dysfunction. Which cardiac conditions in particular should verapamil NOT be given in?
4. Why should verapamil and digoxin as well as diltiazem and digoxin NOT be given together?
5. Why are beta blockers and verapamil administration spaced apart?
6. Grapefruit juice is known to increase toxicity of both of these medications. What are signs of toxicity with verapamil and diltiazem?
7. What is the treatment for both these medications when toxic levels are reached?

Agents that Act Mainly on Vascular Smooth Muscle

Nifedipine

1. Why is nifedipine NOT used for the treatment of cardiac dysrhythmias?
2. What are the therapeutic uses of nifedipine?

Tips for answering exam questions related to these medications (Rosenjack Burchum et al., 2016)

- Nifedipine can cause reflex tachycardia with the immediate-release formulation due to sympathetic nervous stimulation (fall in blood pressure stimulates the sympathetic response)
- Nifedipine has side effects such as gingival hyperplasia and may pose a risk of chronic eczematous rash in older clients
- Reflex tachycardia can be prevented when nifedipine is administered with a beta blocker medication
- Beta blockers can INTENSIFY the effects of verapamil and dilitizem and are NOT typically given together
- Verapamil and diltiazem are contraindicated for clients with severe hypo tension, sick sinus syndrome, second-degree or third-degree AV block
- Calcium channel blockers can also cause peripheral edema

BETA BLOCKERS

Help to treat angina by slowing the heart rate (negative chronotropic effect) and decreasing myocardial contractility (negative inotropic effect). This results in decreasing myocardial oxygen demand (because a rapidly beating heart requires more oxygen) and the negative chronotropic effect increases oxygen delivery to the myocardium. Beta blockers block the beta-adrenergic receptors which are stimulated by the binding of the neurotransmitters epinephrine and norepinephrine. Beta blockers are most effective for exertional angina because they blunt the usual physiological increase in heart rate and systolic BP that occurs during exercise or stress, thereby decreasing myocardial oxygen demand.

In order to understand Beta Blockers fully it is helpful to review physiology of adrenergic receptors. https://www.youtube.com/watch?v=Ip1o57qIoZw

Table 5.4: Types of Beta Blocker Medications

Drug	Pharmacologic Class	Indication
Acebutolol	Beta1-blocker	Hypertension, Angina
Atenolol	Beta1-blocker	Hypertension, Angina
Bisoprolol	Beta1-blocker	Mild to moderate hypertension
Carvedilol	Alpha1- and beta-blocker	Heart Failure
Esmolol	Beta1-blocker	Supraventricular tachydysrhythmias, Intra-operative/post-operative tachycardia and hypertension
Labetalol	Alpha and beta-blocker	Hypertension, Severe hypertension
Metoprolol	Beta1-blocker	Hypertension, late myocardial infarction, early myocardial infarction, angina
Propranolol	Beta-blocker	Prophylaxis for angina, hypertension, post-MI, migraine, serious dysrhythmias
Sotalol	Beta-blocker	Life-threatening ventricular dysrhythmias

1. Identify how beta-blockers work to control hypertension.
2. Why would beta-blockers be used in: myocardial infarction, treatment of angina or dysrhythmia management?
3. Beta-blockers can mask hypoglycemia. How does this occur? Identify how the nurse should assess for hypoglycemia for diabetic clients taking beta-blocker therapy.
4. Identify the difference between selective and non-selective beta blockers. How should the nurse approach beta blocker therapy in a client with asthma in light of this information?
5. What the three most significant side effects associated with beta-blocker therapy?
6. Are there any disease conditions in which beta-blocker therapy is absolutely contraindicated?

Tips for answering exam questions related to these medications (Rosenjack Burchum et al., 2016)

- If a client has a low heart rate as a result of beta blocker therapy always look in the exam question for clues such as blood pressure, level of consciousness, dizziness, etc. to assess how stable they are. Remember, after a myocardial infarction the goal is to reduce the workload of the heart.
- Always think about the indication for beta-blocker therapy when assessing if it is appropriate to give the medication.
- Never give a beta-blocker to a client with a history of sick sinus syndrome or second-or-third-degree AV block. Beta-blockers can be used with care in clients with heart failure.
- The most significant side effects of these medications are: bradycardia, decreased AV conduction and reduced contractility. It is important to understand the client's pathology and if these potential side effects are helpful or harmful to them.
- If a client develops symptomatic bradycardia with beta blocker therapy, they can be changed to the following beta blocker drugs because they don't slow the heart rate at rest as much as the other drugs in this class do: acebutolol, penbutolol, pindolol

ACE INHIBITORS

1. How do ACE Inhibitors work to decrease hypertension and to prevent cardiac remodeling (in the context of heart failure)?
2. Identify four of the most prominent side effects associated with ACE Inhibitors. Identify symptoms associated with each side effect.

Tips for answering exam questions related to these medications (Rosenjack Burchum et al., 2016):

- In hypertensive, diabetic clients these medications slow the progression of kidney disease
- These medications (and beta blockers) are less effective in individuals of African-American descent
- Avoid potassium supplementation or potassium sparing diuretics in clients using ACE Inhibitors
- Do not give ACE Inhibitors to pregnant women as they are proven to cause fetal harm (never indicated for preeclampsia)

ANGIOTENSION II RECEPTOR BLOCKERS

1. How do Angiotension II receptor blockers differ from ACE Inhibitors in their mechanism of action?
2. Can Angiotension II receptor blockers be given to pregnant women experiencing preeclampsia?

3. Angiotension II receptor blockers do not cause a persistent cough or significant hyperkalemia in clients. However, they share one similar side effect to ACE inhibitors, what is it?

NITRATES

Nitroglycerin is used for prophylaxis and treatment of angina and other cardiac problems (Lilley, Harrington, Snyder, Rainforth Collins, S. & Swart, 2010). Nitrates cause both large and small coronary arteries to dilate resulting in a decrease in venous return and a lower left ventricular end-diastolic volume (preload), this results in lower left ventricular pressure and decreases myocardial oxygen demand. Nitrates also alleviate coronary artery spasm (Variant or Prinzmetal's angina). Remember, nitrates vasodilate smooth muscle, when atherosclerotic plaques are complete the vessel cannot be dilated.

1. What are known contraindications to nitrate therapy?
2. What are noted side effects of nitrates? Outline a care plan for treating a client experiencing side effects related to nitroglycerin therapy.
3. Why is reflex tachycardia a concern during nitrate administration?
4. Complete a drug card for isosorbide mononitrate and nitroglycerine (include the dose ranges and routes for the medication).

Tips for answering exam questions related to these medications (Rosenjack Burchum et al., 2016):

- A rare side effect of nitrate administration is **methemoglobinemia** which occurs in clients with an inherent genetic propensity for the condition, iron in hemoglobin is oxidized from the ferrous to the ferric state resulting in an inability to transport oxygen normally—symptoms are headache, fatigue, shortness of breath, potentially shock and seizures.
- When administering nitrate therapy, it is important to examine the entire clinical presentation of the client. Look in the exam question to see which vital signs are provided, the indication for admission or suspected pathology, and what the intended outcome should be. For example, if a client is admitted with angina and requires vasodilation to stop ischemia then nitrate administration would be appropriate. However, if the client has a low blood pressure and a suspected infarct in the right ventricle nitrate administration may not be appropriate at that time.

Cardiac Specific Medications

CARDIAC GLYCOSIDE (Digoxin)

1. What are the indications for digoxin therapy?
2. Outline the necessary assessments prior to the administration of digoxin therapy.
3. Predisposing factors to cardiac dysrhythmias resulting from digoxin administration include: hypokalemia and elevated digoxin levels. Outline why these two factors would cause dysrhythmias.
4. What drug is used in severe digoxin toxicity or overdose?
5. What are the most common GI side effects noted with digoxin toxicity?
6. Digoxin is related to a large number of drug interactions. Complete the following table outlining why these combined drugs may cause digoxin toxicity:

Drug Interaction with Digoxin	How the Drug might Influence Digoxin Levels in the Body or Put Client at Risk for Toxicity
Diuretics (Thiazide & Loop Diuretics)	
ACE Inhibitors and ARBs	
Sympathomimetics (dopamine, dobutamine)—note: pairing these drugs with digoxin can be beneficial but there are some risks	
Quinidine	
Verapamil	

Tips for answering exam questions related to these medications (Rosenjack Burchum et al., 2016):

- Focus on client assessment and recognition of toxicity
- While serum drug levels are taken for digoxin therapy, clients should also be assessed for symptoms of toxicity as well

- Potassium levels are important and any drugs decreasing potassium should be noted so the client can be watched for signs of digoxin toxicity
- Digoxin therapy used to be given in a loading dose to increase high plasma drug levels (digitalization) this is no longer the practice. It takes 6 days to achieve plasma levels without a loading dose.

ANTIDYSRHYTHMIC MEDICATIONS

1. Draw out the Cardiac Action Potential (phases 0-4) and outline what happens in each phase
2. In the table below, input where Class I-IV agents work during the cardiac action potential
3. Adverse effects are significant in this type of drug therapy. Make a drug card for medications in each of the classes outlined in the table below (these represent the most common medications given in each class).

Table 5.5 Indications for Antidysrhythmic Drugs

Class I: Sodium Channel Blockers	Long term suppression of ventricular and supraventricular dysrhythmias
Class 1a agents (quinidine, procainamide, disopyramide)	Atrial fibrillation, premature atrial contractions, premature ventricular contractions, sustained ventricular tachycardia
Class Ib agents (lidocaine, phenytoin)	Ventricular dysrhythmias only (premature ventricular contractions, v-tach, v-fib)
Class Ic (flecainide & propafenone)	Severe ventricular dysrhythmias only may use in a-fib/a-flutter
Class II agents beta blockers (propranolol)	General myocardial depressants for both supraventricular and ventricular dysrhythmias
Class III agents (amiodarone, dronedarone, sotalol)	Life-threatening ventricular tachycardia or fibrillation Atrial fibrillation or flutter in acute settings
Class IV agents (Calcium Channel Blockers)- diltiazem & verapamil	Paroxysmal supraventricular tachycardia; rate control for atrial fibrillation and flutter
Others: Adenosine	Paroxysmal supraventricular tachycardia

The remaining questions in this section focus on life-threatening or unique side effects related to anti-dysrhythmic medications.

1. Cinchonism may occur in clients receiving Quinidine therapy. What is this condition?
2. Cardiotoxicity is a common side effect related to antidysrhythmic medications. What is this and how is it clinically identified?
3. Quinidine can double digoxin levels. What are signs of digoxin toxicity?
4. A client is being switched from IV to po procainamide. How much time should be between stopping the IV infusion and administering the first oral dose?
5. SLE-like syndrome is associated with procainamide, what are signs of this side effect? If the client is unable to discontinue procainamide due to the complexity of their condition, how is SLE-like syndrome treated?
6. Blood dyscrasias such as agranulocytosis, thrombocytopenia and neutropenia can occur in clients receiving procainamide. What are signs and symptoms of these conditions?
7. What can happen if a client is given excessive doses of lidocaine?
8. Amiodarone is a medication that can potentially cause pulmonary toxicity, cardiac toxicity, liver toxicity, thyroid toxicity, and toxicity in pregnancy and breast-feeding. Identify clinical signs of toxicity due to amiodarone therapy in each of these areas.
9. Amiodarone can also cause skin discolouration. What colour does it turn the skin after prolonged use?
10. Amiodarone has multiple drug-to-drug interactions. Identify which drugs: 1) can have their levels increased by amiodarone therapy, 2) drugs that can reduce amiodarone levels, 3) drugs that can increase the risk of dysrhythmias when given with amiodarone and 4) drugs that can cause excessive bradycardia when given with amiodarone.
11. Identify the mechanism of action of adenosine. What specific teaching would the nurse provide to the client when administering this medication?

Drugs to Reduce Cardiac Risk Factors

HMG-CoA REDUCTASE INHIBITORS

1. Myopathy/Rhabdomyolysis is a potential side effect occurring with the use of statin medications. What are symptoms of this condition and how is it treated?
2. Niacin reduces LDL and TG levels, while increasing HDL better than any other drug. However, it does little to improve outcomes (p. 571). What are some frequent side effects associated with this medication?
3. Flushing is a side effect of Niacin administration. What should the nurse advise the client to take 30 minutes prior to administering a dose of Niacin to counteract this frequent side effect?

4. Are bile-acid sequestrants absorbed by the GI tract? How does this influence systemic absorption of these medications?
5. Bile-acid sequestrants can form insoluable complexes with other drugs, thereby severely limiting their absorption. Which medications are known to form complexes with bile-acid sequestrants?
6. Create a drug cards for ezetimibe and gemfibrozil. Which drugs does it potentially act with these medications? Why are clients taking this medication at an increased risk of gallstones?

Tips for answering exam questions related to these medications (Rosenjack Burchum et al., 2016, p. 570-571)

- When statin drugs are combined with other lipid-lowering agents use extra caution and monitor for adverse effects more frequently.
- If the goal is to lower LDL cholesterol 30-40% then any type of statin drug is recommended, if LDL must be lowered by 40% or higher atorvastatin or simvastatin may be preferred.
- If a client has renal impairment atorvastatin and fluvastatin are preferred (because no dose adjustment is needed).
- For medications that are known to form insoluble complexes with bile-acid sequestrants, how long should they be administered between each other so complexes do not occur?
- Bile-acid sequestrants should be mixed with water, fruit juice, soup or pulpy fruit to reduce esophageal irritation and impaction.

ANTICOAGULANT/ANTIPLATELET/THROMBOLYTIC THERAPY

Table 5.3 outlines all the drug classes of anticoagulant/antiplatelet and thrombolytic drugs. The review questions below focus on the most common medications given. It is recommended for drug classes such as glycoprotein IIb/IIIa Receptor Antagonists, Direct Thrombin Inhibitors, Direct Factor Xa Inhibitors and Antithrombin drugs that you **choose the most common drug out of each class and make a drug card for it**. The other drug classes contain medications that you may have more commonly administered in your clinical practice to date. The review questions below focus on pulling out more detailed information from these common drug classes.

1. What is the antidote for Warfarin? Do the other oral anticoagulants: rivaroxaban, apixaban & dabigatran have antidotes?
2. What baseline blood values should be taken prior to administering heparin therapy?
3. How much should aPTT increase for heparin to be effective?
4. Describe Heparin-Induced Thrombocytopenia and how it is treated.
5. Identify conditions in which warfarin is absolutely contraindicated for.
6. What are common drug-to-drug interactions involving warfarin?
7. Can clopidogrel and aspirin be administered concurrently?

8. Create a teaching plan outlining: 1) signs of bleeding and 2) when to contact the health care provider when taking any type of anticoagulant therapy.
9. What is thrombotic thrombocytopenic purpura (TTP)? Which anticoagulant medications is this potential side effect associated with?
10. Review conditions that would be absolute contraindications for thrombolytic therapy. Which clients would meet the criteria for administration with great caution?

Tips for answering exam questions related to these medications (Rosenjack Burchum et al., 2016):

- Warfarin's dose is adjusted based on INR and requires blood sampling; however, doses for rivaroxaban, apixaban & dabigatran etexilate are fixed and do not require blood tests.
- Avoid high-dose therapy of anticoagulant and antiplatelet medications when a thrombolytic drug is being administered.

Integrative Therapy Caution

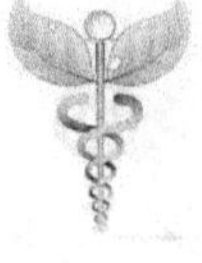

Herbal Medication: Green Tea

Dried green tea leaves contain Vitamin K and large amounts may interfere with warfarin. Decrease in INR has been reported with green tea (Richards, 2013).

Integrative Therapy Caution

Herbal Medication: Ginger

Used primarily for nausea and vomiting during pregnancy (under supervision of HCP), treatment and prevention of motion sickness, vertigo and to increase appetite and reduce stomach acidity. Ginger can prolong bleeding time and may cause interactions with warfarin, ASA, and other blood thinners (Richards, 2013).

Table 5.6: Summary of Different Indications for Cardiac Medications

Drug Name	Mechanism of Action	Indications for Angina	Indications for Myocardial Infarction (MI)	Indications for Heart Failure	Indications for Dysrhythmias
Nitrates Routes: SL, IV, spray, patch Contraindicated: Aortic stenosis, pericardial tamponade, constrictive pericarditis (p.292) Do NOT give with: alcohol (monitor use: causes further hypotension), Viagra (within 24 hours of last dose), caution with glaucoma, caution with severe liver , kidney disease or early MI.	• Relaxes both arterial and venous smooth muscle • Dilates coronary arteries • Decreases preload • Reduces cardiac output/ workload of heart decreased • Lowers myocardial oxygen demand Short acting: nitroglycerin Long acting: isosorbide dinitrate **Tolerance may develop* **Monitor**: - BP and pulse prior to administration. **May cause reflex tachycardia and hypotension.* - Always reassess pain and need for medication	-Once thought to dilate only the coronary arteries, nitrates are now primarily given to decrease preload and myocardial oxygen demand during angina. -Relieves chest pain (goal is 0/10 level of chest pain) -Always do 12 lead ECG and assess for hypotension prior to giving - May cause headache Nitroglycerin most common nitrate given for angina.	-Given to vasodilate coronary arteries, reduce cardiac output and demand and lower myocardial oxygen demand. Give with caution in patients experiencing acute myocardial infarction and decreased preload: may further extend area of infarct. -Given IV during unstable angina and MI (if not contraindicated) if pain not controlled. Nitroglycerin most common nitrate given during MI.	Play a minor role in HF. Isosorbide dinitrate given in HF to relax blood vessels and lower blood pressure. Acts directly on the veins. Generally reserved for patients who cannot tolerate ACE Inhibitors. Isosorbide dinitrate and hydralazine are often paired together for treatment.	NOT INDICATED

Drug Name	Mechanism of Action	Indications for Angina	Indications for Myocardial Infarction (MI)	Indications for Heart Failure	Indications for Dysrhythmias
Beta-Blockers Contraindicated: Bradycardia, second and third degree heart block, decompensated HF, and cardiogenic shock Use with caution: Asthma, COPD, impaired renal function In diabetics may mask signs of hypoglycemia *See prototype in module of* ***carvedilol (a*** *non-selective BB)*	• Blocks catecholamines • Reduces the workload of the heart (negative chronotropic effect) • Reduces contractility (negative inotropic effect) • Tolerance does not develop • Used for angina, MI, dysrhythmias and hypertension **Assess and monitor:** pulse rate, blood pressure, shortness of breath and respiratory distress (usually in pts with asthma) Do not abruptly discontinue as excitation of adrenergic receptors may occur: causing angina, tachycardia, or MI. **Common beta blockers:** metoprolol, atenolol, propanolol. $Beta_1$ blockers will NOT affect lungs (also referred to as selective BB) Metoprolol most common.	- First line drug for chronic stable angina - Decreases the frequency and severity of angina attacks caused by exertion - Decreases workload of the heart and prevent myocardial ischemia to some degree - Do not give with HR below 50.	Slow heart rate, decrease contractility, and reduce blood pressure Thereby reduces myocardial oxygen demand Slow impulse conduction through the heart, which suppresses dysrhythmias Shown to reduce mortality when given 8 hours after onset of MI Do not give with HR below 50.	Reduce cardiac workload; HF causes excessive activation of SNA, which weakens the heart and leads to progression of HF. Beta blockers inhibit these SNS effects. Slows heart rate and reduces blood pressure. Thereby decreasing afterload. Do not give with HR below 50. Therapy may normalize heart size, shape and function in some patients. Must be started on very low doses. Expect these doses to be 1/10 of what you would use in angina or MI. Initial high doses may worsen HF. Never used alone for HF, always paired with ACE inhibitors. Always report worsening symptoms of HF (weight gain, edema, SOB) as dose may be causing this	Class II antidysrhythmic drug Slows heart rate and conduction velocity through the AV node to suppress several types of dysrhythmias Used to treat atrial dysrhythmias in pts with HF Abrupt discontinuation may cause hypotension and dysrhythmias Do not give with HR below 50

Drug Name	Mechanism of Action	Indications for Angina	Indications for Myocardial Infarction (MI)	Indications for Heart Failure	Indications for Dysrhythmias
Calcium Channel Blockers (CCB) Contraindicated: Sick sinus syndrome or third degree AV block without presence of pacemaker; severe hypotension Use with caution: May worsen HF by decreasing myocardial contractility; avoid grapefruit juice may elevate drug to toxic levels. May cause edema, shortness of breath—take pulse frequently if falls below 60. Take BP freq.	May be used in pts who cannot tolerate BB; CCB may also be combined with BB in pts with persistent symptoms • Inhibits flow of Ca into smooth muscle • Relaxes arteriolar smooth muscle • Causes peripheral vascular dilation • Reduces afterload, and myocardial oxygen demand • Slows conduction velocity through the heart • Dilates coronary arteries and relieve vasospasm **Dihydropyridine CCB:** amlodipine and nifedipine (may combine with beta-blockers) **Non-dihydropyridine CCB:** Verapamil and diltiazem (do not combine with beta-blockers: has effects on conduction)	Amlodipine and nifedipine relax arteriolar smooth muscle and lower blood pressure, reducing afterload and reducing myocardial demand. Verapamil and diltiazem relax arteriolar smooth muscle and also slow conduction velocity through the heart, decreasing HR and reducing myocardial demand CCB dilate coronary arteries and relive acute vasospasm (variant angina)	May be given for coronary vasospasm or hypertension. Given for other symptoms in order to increase myocardial oxygen. May be an option if pts cannot tolerate beta blocker therapy.	CCB may be given for pts who cannot take BB therapy. However, they may worsen heart failure. Use with caution in patients with severe heart failure.	Only a limited number of CCB have been approved to treat dysrhythmias Reduce automaticity in the SA node and slow impulse conduction through the AV node Prolongs refractory period and stabilizes many types of dysrhythmias. Only effective against supraventricular dysrhythmias. Sometimes these actions may cause pts with existing heart abnormalities to experience adverse events: Calcium chloride slow IV push may reverse hypotension or heart block induced by CCB. Educate pt to inform nurse if heart feels like it is "skipping beats".

Drug Name	Mechanism of Action	Indications for Angina	Indications for Myocardial Infarction (MI)	Indications for Heart Failure	Indications for Dysrhythmias
ACE Inhibitors **Use with caution:** impaired kidney function, hyperkalemia, autoimmune diseases. May cause neutropenia, may increase creatinine 30% when initiated. Discontinue diuretics when they are first initiated to prevent hypotension. May cause angioedema: expected after onset of therapy and then resolves. If it persists, inform physician.	• Inhibits the formation of angiotension II • Reduces afterload of the heart and lower blood pressure • Lowers blood pressure by action on renin-angiotension aldosterone system • Inhibits aldosterone excretion • Increases cardiac output • Dilates veins returning blood to the heart, also reduces preload and reduces edema. **Monitor:** BP and electrolytes Therapeutic effects may take weeks or months for maximum effects. **Dietary modifications**: Na and K restrictions. May cause hyperkalemia	Not given to patients with angina unless they are already receiving the ACE Inhibitor for hypertension, previous MI, or HF	Shown to reduce mortality in pts with MI if administered soon after onset of symptoms	Drugs of choice in the treatment of HF. Used to prevent HF for those at risk and slow the progression of HF in those that have it. Helps the heart for all of the reasons listed on the bullet points under "Mechanisms of Action" Replace digoxin as the drug of choice for tx of HF	Not indicated for dysrhythmias

Drug Name	Mechanism of Action	Indications for Angina	Indications for Myocardial Infarction (MI)	Indications for Heart Failure	Indications for ysrhythmias
Cardiac Glycosides (e.g., Digoxin) Evaluate for: previous ventricular dysrhythmias not caused by HF, any history of hypersensitivity, renal impairment, incomplete heart block.	• Reserved for pts whose symptoms persist despite the use of first line drugs • Inhibits Na, K –ATPase, which is responsible for pumping Na out of the cell in exchange for a K+ ion. As Na accumulates, Ca+ ions are released into the cell producing a more forceful contraction of myocardial fibers. • Causes heart to beat more forcefully and more slowly, increasing cardiac output • Narrow therapeutic index; must monitor levels closely through blood work	NOT INDICATED	NOT INDICATED	Increases cardiac output, alleviating symptoms of HF and improves exercise tolerance. Results in increased urine production and a reduction in blood volume, relieving pulmonary congestion and peripheral edema.	Has the ability to suppress SA node and slow electrical conduction through the AV node. Given for atrial dysrhythmias. Common for dysrhythmias to occur when high doses of digoxin are administered. Can give Digibind in this case to block the action of digoxin. **Digoxin toxicity:** Symptoms include fatigue, nausea/vomiting, changes in heart rate and rhythm, loss of appetite (anorexia), diarrhea, visual disturbances (yellow or green halos around objects), confusion, dizziness, nightmares, agitation, and/or depression, as well as sensory reactions.

Drug Name	Mechanism of Action	Indications for Angina	Indications for Myocardial Infarction (MI)	Indications for Heart Failure	Indications for Dysrhythmias
Diuretic Therapy Contraindicated in: Renal failure, pregnancy, fluid and electrolyte depletion and hepatic coma **Evaluate for**: Potassium levels, weakness, hypotension and confusion, monitor electrolytes, BUN, hyperglycemia and anemia	• Reduce blood volume, edema and pulmonary congestion • Reduces the workload of the heart • Increases cardiac output • Often prescribed with ACE Inhibitors or other HF drugs **Monitor**: V/S, intake and output. Rapid diuresis can result in dehydration, hypovolemia and circulatory collapse. Monitor daily Na intake, report weight loss of more than 1kg per week, report fatigue and muscle cramping, change positions slowly as dizziness may occur in combination with other drug therapy.	NOT INDICATED	NOT INDICATED	Most common medication for acute heart failure: Furosemide (Lasix). Important note do not give this drug with digoxin will cause dysrhythmias. Other diuretics may be given once pt is stabilized or if they are dealing with chronic heart failure. Diuretic regime is often dependent on other co-morbidities and extent of heart failure.	NOT INDICATED

Drug Name	Mechanism of Action	Indications for Angina	Indications for Myocardial Infarction (MI)	Indications for Heart Failure	Indications for Dysrhythmias
Antiplatelets **Evaluate for**: Thrombocytopenia, Bleeding, increased risk of bleeding if ASA, given with other NSAIDS	• Prevents platelet aggregation and clot formation. Please review the mechanism of action of the following drugs separately: 1. ASA 2. Clopidogrel (Plavix) 3. Glycoprotein IIb/IIIa inhibitors • Remember that although heparin is often given in conjunction with these medications, it is an anticoagulant drug, *not* an antiplatelet. Therefore, if a patient is receiving both, they must be monitored closely.	ASA may be given as prophylactic therapy for individuals with angina, or unstable angina. Clopidogrel (Plavix) is also given to prevent MI. Also given as a loading dose prior to angioplasty, then pt is put on daily dose of medication	160-325 mg of ASA is given as soon as MI is suspected. **ASA** is used in weeks following acute MI to decrease pt mortality. **Clopidogrel** (Plavix) and **ticlopidine (Ticlid)** are used for the prevention of thromobotic stroke and MI. They block adenosine diphosphate. More expensive than ASA; usually for pts allergic to ASA or at a greater risk of GI bleed from ASA. **Glycoprotein IIb/IIIa inhibitors**: Occupy receptor sites on platelets and inhibit clot formation. Often used for unstable angina, MI or PTCA.	NOT INDICATED—*should not be given if there is a history of CAD or previous MI. But antiplatelets do NOT treat heart failure*	NOT INDICATED

Drug Name	Mechanism of Action	Indications for Angina	Indications for Myocardial Infarction (MI)	Indications for Heart Failure	Indications for Dysrhythmias
Thrombolytics or Fibrinolytic therapy **Contraindicated in**: recent trauma, surgery, biopsy, arterial emboli, cerebral embolism, hemorrhage, thrombo-cytopenia, septic thrombo-phlebitis or childbirth (within 10 days)	• Dissolves blood clots in the coronary arteries. • Converts plasminogen to plasmin, the enzyme plasmin digests fibrin and breaks down fibrinogen, prothrombin and other plasma proteins and clotting factors. • Has a narrow margin of safety. **Monitor**: V/S monitored closely; monitor for any signs of bleeding; take a thorough patient history ensuring there is no PUD; hx of bleeding or recent surgery	NOT INDICATED	Give within 4 hours of onset of MI symptoms. Ideal to give ASAP first 20-40 minutes after onset of symptoms. Common drugs given: TPA: Tissue plasminogen activator TNK- t-pa: Tenecteplase Streptokinase (not used as often) Obtain baseline PT and aPTT prior to initiating therapy, as well as CBC Start 2 IV lines, arterial line, and Foley catheter prior to administering Assess for changes in level of consciousness and check neurological status, since cerebral hemorrhage is a major concern In MI, dysrhythmias may result when the clot is destroyed and tissue perfusion occurs. Often they are benign and resolve on their own	NOT INDICATED	NOT INDICATED

Integrative Therapy Caution

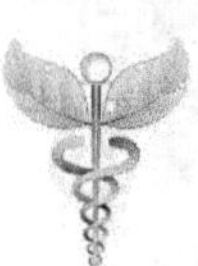

Herbal Medication: Feverfew

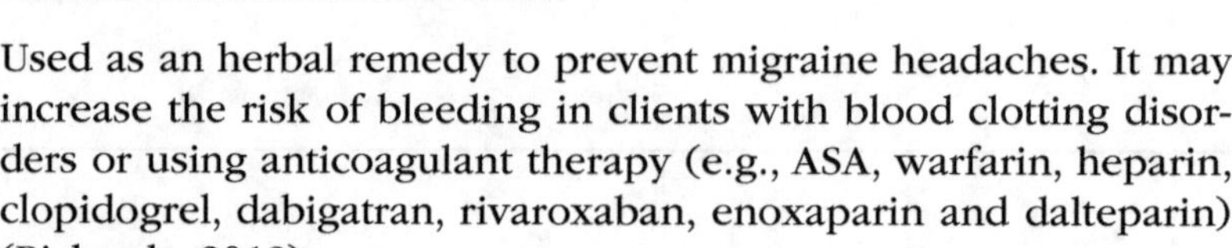

Used as an herbal remedy to prevent migraine headaches. It may increase the risk of bleeding in clients with blood clotting disorders or using anticoagulant therapy (e.g., ASA, warfarin, heparin, clopidogrel, dabigatran, rivaroxaban, enoxaparin and dalteparin) (Richards, 2013).

PRACTICE QUESTIONS

Question 1
A client is taking nifedipine for angina pectoris. The client has a known history of heart failure and AV conduction delay. Recently the client has been experiencing reflex tachycardia related to drug therapy. Which directive should the nurse expect the Health Care Provider to order to combat this side effect of this medication?

1. Administer Metoprolol 25 mg po bid and continue nifedipine therapy
2. Discontinue nifedipine therapy and start verapamil 120mg SR capsules daily
3. Administer atropine 1mg sc immediately
4. Discontinue nifedipine therapy and administer nitroglycerin 0.4mg transdermal patch daily

Question 2
A pregnant woman has been diagnosed with preeclampsia and requires medication to treat her hypertension. She has been admitted to a tertiary care centre and delivering the baby is currently not an option due to early gestation. What is the expected drug therapy for this condition?

1. Ramipril 2.5mg po bid
2. Metoprolol 25mpg po daily
3. Furosemide 20mg IV direct
4. Labetalol 20mg IV bolus over 2 minutes

Question 3
A client has been started on rivaroxaban. What should the nurse teach the client receiving this medication?

1. INR monitoring is not required for this drug therapy
2. Frequent INR monitoring is required for this drug therapy
3. Side effects such as excessive blood clotting can occur
4. Frequent aPTT monitoring is recommended for this medication

Question 4
A client taking nitroglycerin therapy has a genetic predisposition to developing **methemoglobinemia**. What are prominent symptoms of this condition? **(Select all that apply)**

1. Headache
2. Fatigue
3. Shortness of breath
4. Excessive diuresis
5. Seizures

Question 5

A client receiving procainamide for long-term management of supraventricular dysrhythmias has developed SLE-like syndrome. Which of the following assessment findings should the nurse expect to find in a client with this side effect of procainamide therapy? **(Select all that apply)**

1. Joint pain and inflammation
2. Unexplained fever
3. Decreased urine output
4. Increased incidences of bleeding
5. Soreness of mouth, throat or gums

Question 6

A client with type 2 diabetes is receiving metoprolol 25 mg po daily after a myocardial infarction. Due to uncontrolled blood glucose levels the client is also started on aspart insulin via insulin pen prior to meals. What is a priority area for client education for this client?

1. Instruct the client to wash their skin with soap and water prior to injecting the insulin
2. Teach the client that insulin aspart is an intermediate acting insulin
3. Teach the client to monitor their blood glucose levels closely because hypoglycemia may be masked
4. Instruct the client to take their heart rate prior to taking metoprolol each morning

Answers: Question 1(1), Question 2(4), Question 3 (1), Question 4(1,2,3,5), Question 5(1,2,5), Question 6 (3)

Study Strategy

This study guide differs from other resources because formal rationale is not provided for the answers. **You need to determine the appropriate rationale for the correct answers by accessing the information in the question that may have inhibited your ability to answer the question correctly.** It is helpful to ask the following questions:

- What is the question asking? What are key words in the question query?
- What information do I need to know to answer this question correctly?
- How did I select my answer?
- Why were the other answers incorrect?
- Was I missing a piece of content knowledge that inhibited how I answered the question? If so, what should I target in on and study?

Additional Strategies for Working with the Pharmacology Study Guide Modules

Content review is essential for being successful at answering NCLEX-RN® exam questions focusing on pharmacology. The following tips will help you to navigate the breath of this content and to organize your study notes. **Remember that you need to do the work of solid content review in order to be successful in understanding pharmacological concepts. Do not rely on practice questions to teach you what you need to know regarding medications for the NCLEX-RN®- practice questions are a tool for consolidating knowledge not a primary way to study.**

1. Complete the exercises in this study guide and make notes. This guide has been designed to direct you to important content for medication review. When creating the study guide I used an educator's lens to pull out the most important information in order ensure client safety with drug administration. For example, when review differing drugs I focused on critical information and essential education for each drug. The review questions are designed to bring this information forward.
2. Find ways to colour code or organize medications according to the bodily system or pathology they are used for. This will help you with recalling information. This guide uses a systems approach to help you organize the vast amount of pharmacological review in a way that will help you understand key concepts and pathologies.
3. Create case studies or unique ways to remember classes of medications. It is always wise to study pharmacology in the context of pathology. Use case studies specifically for content that is new to you or more difficult. Case studies should be memorable, contain client information that is easy to remember, focus on adverse effects of medications and key aspects of client education.
4. It is helpful to find patterns in names in drugs- such as suffixes that are common. Highlight the endings of common terms and find strategies to remember the main side effects of these classes of medications.
5. Client teaching is essential in medication administration. Ensure that you review your client education chapter in your Fundamentals of Nursing textbook (e.g. Potter and Perry). You need to remember that the use of basic teaching and learning principles paired with your knowledge of medications can help you to better exam questions.
6. When you use practice questions find consistent strategies for reviewing questions that you get incorrect. For example, the summary drug tables presented in each module of this guide provide a structure for organizing information. Create a blank table with the drug classes named for each system. Write information or content that is tested in each drug class as you move through your practice resources. Highlight the medication names you have seen in the practice questions on your summary table. Are there any

patterns in the types of questions asked or the content tested? **Do be careful with this strategy- it is not a replacement for reviewing content.**

Conclusion

Strong pharmacological review will not only increase your chances of success on the NCLEX-RN® it will also strengthen your future nursing practice. The complexity of client care paired with the increase in co-morbidity and chronic disease management poses many challenges to pharmacological therapy. Nurses must be aware of potential drug-to-drug interactions, polypharmacy, and adverse events related to medications in order to keep their clients safe. I wish you all the best for your NCLEX-RN® exam and for your future nursing practice.

Best wishes,
Dr. Marnie Kramer-Kile

REFERENCES

Copstead, L.E & Banaski, J. (2013). *Pathophysiology* (5th ed). St. Louis: Elsevier.

Richards, J.S. (2013). Overview of herbal supplements. *Elite Continuing Education,* 46-72.

Rosenjack Burchum, J. & Rosenthal, L.D. (2016). *Lehne's pharmacology for nursing care* (9th edition). St. Louis: Elsevier.

Module 6

Drugs Affecting the Urinary and Renal System

TABLE OF CONTENTS

Tables and Figures

Introduction to the Transitioning to the NCLEX-RN® Pharmacology Guide: Drugs Affecting the Renal System

The breadth and detail of the knowledge required of pharmacological concepts often overwhelms new graduates when they are beginning their exam preparation. The purpose of this pharmacology study guide is to help you work through the vast amount of pharmacological knowledge required for the NCLEX-RN® in a systematic and purposeful way. This guide organizes content using the current NCLEX-RN® Test Plan and provides specific strategies to address pharmacological areas of review which may challenge new graduates. **This is the sixth of twelve modules.** This is a working guide, so while key information will be presented and organized for review, it is up to you to do the detailed work of content review by answering the questions and exercises in each section. You can expect to see drugs described by their generic names on the exam. Due to the differences in drug trade names between the United States of America, Canada and other countries you should study drugs according to their generic names and develop strategies for remembering them.

This module is part of a comprehensive pharmacology study guide focusing on specific areas which may challenge NCLEX-RN® candidates. This includes drug-to-drug interactions, specific adverse reactions due to drug therapy and the potential reactions associated with herbal therapy and conventional medications. The content will be focused on a systems approach and will direct you towards important information within each drug class.

Structure of the Module

This module begins with an overview of the differing drug classes for the renal system. Additional areas for review that are specialized or affect multiple systems will also be highlighted:

1. Review questions and selected exercises will be constructed for each drug class to help pull out key concepts such as adverse events/side effects, specific client teaching and drug to drug interactions.
2. A summary chart of the drug classes in each system or theme will be provided for you to use alongside practice questions. As you move through practice questions, check off the specific medications you come across and if you require further review in each area. It is also helpful to make your own drug cards for specific medications. Keep the drug cards simple. Identify the drug class, the mechanism of action, two relevant (i.e., life threatening) or unique adverse effects that require monitoring and provide an outline for client teaching or specific nursing interventions for the medication.

Advice for Studying Pharmacological Content for the NCLEX-RN®

Always start with areas you are NOT familiar with. For example, if you spent the majority of your time as a final practicum student/or nurse on a cardiology unit do not start in the Vascular and Cardiac Medications Module. It is common for students/graduates to move to areas of comfort when they are studying because it decreases their anxiety. However, your efforts should be targeted on what you don't know. Each Module in this guide has a summary table of drugs for each system. Highlight the drug classes that you are not familiar with and make it your priority to work through them. Do not spend time making drug cards for medications you already know. For example, most students are confident with furosemide administration and can critically think through concepts associated with the drug. Therefore, time does not need to be spent studying this medication. Only make drug cards for medications that are new to you. The review questions in this guide will direct you towards more detailed information of the medications that you are familiar with and focus on potential areas where exam questions may be asked.

This guide is set up using a **systems approach** for the following reasons: 1) most pharmacology textbooks use this approach to structure content so it will be easier to find the information you need to answer the review questions; 2) using a systems approach allows you to find commonalties in the side effects of drugs influencing a specific system, so you will see patterns arising as you work through this guide; and 3) a systems approach allows for the creation of overall drug summary tables, which will be included in each module of the guide and will provide you with a general sense of the medications you need to cover.

The following resources will aid you in answering questions posed in this guide. This includes:

1. **A pharmacology textbook.** This resource will contain more detailed information pertaining to drug classes and outline general nursing considerations for therapy. I have referenced a pharmacology textbook throughout the writing of this guide.
2. **A drug guide**. These are the guides commonly used for your clinical practice. These resources contain alphabetized drug information. Most importantly, they outline specific pharmacokinetic and pharmacodynamics properties of drugs. You will find information related to drug excretion, protein binding, and therapeutic index in these guides.
3. **An online drug repository** for more detailed information that may not be found in the two resources above. Sometimes it is difficult to find therapeutic index and protein binding for a drug. I have found the following website helpful for this: http://www.drugbank.ca/drugs

Module 6: Drugs Affecting the Urinary and Renal System

Table 6.1: Diuretic Therapy and Drugs for Renal Failure

Loop Diuretics Bumetanide (Bumex) Ethacrynic acid (Edecrin) Furosemide (Lasix) Torsemide (Demadex) **Noted Side Effects:** Serious hypokalemia, blood dysracsias, dehydration, ototoxicity, electrolyte imbalances, circulatory collapse **Potassium-sparing Diuretics** Amiloride hydrochloride (Midamor) Eplerenone (Inspra) Spironolactone (Aldactone) Triamterne (Dyrenium) **Noted Side Effects:** Dysrhythmias (from hyperkalemia), dehydration, hyponatremia, agranulocytosis and other blood dyscrasias	**Thiazide Diuretics** Chlorothiazide (Diuril) Hydochlorothiazide (HydroDIURIL, HCTZ) Bendroflumethiazide (Naturetin) Benzthiazide (Aquatage, Exna, Hydrex) Hydroflumethiazide (Diucardin, Saluron) Metolazone (Zaroxolyn, Mykrox) Quinethazone (Hydromax) Chlorthalidone (Hygroton) Inapamide (Lozol) Methyclothiazide (Aquatensen, Enduron) Polythiazide (Renese) Trichlormethiazide (Metahydrin, Naqua, Niazide, Diurese) **Noted Side Effects**: serious hypokalemia, electrolyte depletion, dehydration, hypotension, hyponatremia, hyperglycemia, coma, blood dyscrasias
Miscellaneous Diuretics **Carbonic Anhydrase Inhibitors** Acetazolamide (Diamox) Dichlorphenamide (Darnide, Oratrol) Methazolamide (Neptazane)	**Osmotic** Mannitol (osmitrol) Urea (Ureaphil)

Most diuretics work by blocking sodium and chloride reabsorption, this action creates osmotic pressure in the nephron that prevents the passive reabsorption of water (Rosenjack Burchum et al., 2016, p. 450), thereby causing water and solutes to be contained in the nephron where they are excreted. The amount of urine flow (urine lost) is dependent on the amount of sodium and chloride that are blocked in the nephron. Therefore, drugs that act in the proximal part of the nephron block the largest amount solute reabsorption and thereby have the greatest effects towards diuresis. Drugs that act on the distal part of the nephron have little diuresis. Due to the action of diuretics they will have **3 adverse reactions on extracellular fluid** because they interfere with the normal action of the kidneys (Rosenjack Burchum et al., 2016, p. 450):

1. Hypovolemia (excessive fluid loss)
2. Acid-base imbalance
3. Altered electrolyte levels

REVIEW QUESTIONS

LOOP DIURETICS

1. What is the onset of action of IV furosemide, and when would this route be indicated for a client? Identify conditions that would justify the use of furosemide over other classes of diuretics.
2. Why is furosemide often useful in clients with renal impairment?
3. Describe how the nurse would assess for the following complications related to furosemide therapy: hyponatremia, hypochloremia, dehydration, hypotension, hypokalemia, ototoxicity, hyperglycemia (not common, but due to inhibition of insulin release), hyperuricemia.
4. Identify other ototoxic drugs that may combine with furosemide to increase chances of ototoxicity.
5. Which specific lab value should be monitored closely if a client is receiving digoxin and furosemide?
6. What risks are associated with giving furosemide and lithium concurrently?
7. Why do NSAIDS blunt the effects of furosemide?

Tips for answering exam questions related to these medications (Rosenjack Burchum et al., 2016):

- Loop diuretics are given to clients with low GFR
- Hearing loss is a common side effect of these medications
- Hypokalemia, dehydration, hyperglycemia and hyperuricemia are serious adverse effects
- Always look at the data provided in the exam question to decipher where your focus of assessment should be (e.g., low blood pressure, elevated blood glucose level, increased BUN and client's overall indication for the therapy)

THIAZIDE AND RELATED DIURETICS

1. The ability of thiazide diuretics is contingent on renal function. How low can the GFR go before these drugs are ineffective?
2. How long does it take these drugs to promote diuresis? (use hydrochlorothiazide as your prototype drug)
3. What are the therapeutic uses for these medications?
4. Thiazide diuretics have similar adverse effects to loop diuretics, with some exceptions. What are they?

Tips for answering exam questions related to these medications (Rosenjack Burchum et al., 2016):

- This class of medications reduces blood volume and reduces arterial resistance (this occurs over time and produces long-term effects)
- Hydrochlorothiazide is most widely used
- Hypokalemia is common with these medications. Focus on studying diet plans to increase potassium intake (target specific foods containing potassium)
- Dehydration, hyperglycemia and hyperuricemia are also common adverse effects

POTASSIUM-SPARING DIURETICS

1. In the US, only one aldosterone antagonist is used (spironolactone) and two nonaldosterone antagonists (triamterene & amiloride) are employed. Create drug cards for these medications.
2. What are agents that may increase potassium levels and should be used with caution when administering potassium-sparing diuretics?
3. Spironolactone is a steroid derivative with a structure similar to hormones such as progesterone, estradiol and testosterone. What potential endocrine effects can it cause?

Tips for answering exam questions related to these medications (Rosenjack Burchum et al., 2016, p. 505, 507)

- Degree of diuresis of these medications is small and are often used to balance the hypokalemia caused by other diuretics
- If used alone they can cause hyperkalemia—ensure that clients are not taking potassium supplements
- Do not use these medications routinely with ACE Inhibitors, ARBs or aldosterone antagonists because they promote hyperkalemia

MANNITOL (OSMOTIC DIURETIC)

1. What is the mechanism of action of mannitol? What are the therapeutic uses of this medication?
2. Why is edema an adverse effect of this medication, given that it is a diuretic? Explain the mechanism behind this side effect.
3. If urine flow declines to a very low rate or ceases entirely, the mannitol infusion should be stopped. Why?

Tips for answering exam questions related to these medications (Rosenjack Burchum et al., 2016):

- Mannitol is only given parentally via IV injection
- Mannitol can preserve urine flow and may thereby prevent renal failure
- Mannitol cannot exit the capillary beds of the brain therefore water is kept in the vascular system and then excreted
- In areas other than the brain, mannitol can exit the capillary beds and draws water with it, thereby causing edema. Therefore, this drug is used with caution in clients with CHF.
- Serum osmolality should be monitored when giving this medication

Table 6.2: Other Drugs Influencing the Urinary System

Anticholinergic Drugs for Overactive Bladder (urge incontinence) Darifenacin Oxybutynin Solifenacin Fesoterodine Tolterodine Trospium **These 6 drugs are approved in the USA*	**Drugs to Treat Urinary Retention** Bethanechol	**Treatment of Bladder Spasms** Oxybutynin chloride Tolterodine
<u>Drugs for Acute Cystitis</u> **First-Line Drugs** Trimethoprim/ sulfamethoxazole Nitrofurantoin Fosfomycin **Second-Line Drugs** Ciprofloxacin Levofloxacin	**<u>Drugs for Uncomplicated Pyelonephritis</u>** **First-Line Drugs** Trimethoprim/ sulfamethoxazole Ciprofloxacin Levofloxacin **Second-Line Drugs** Amoxicillin (with clavulanic acid) Cephalexin Cefotaxime Cetriaxone	**Complicated Urinary Tract Infections** Trimethoprim/ sulfamethoxazole Ciprofloxacin Levofloxacin Amoxicillin (with clavulanic acid) Cephalexin **Prophylaxis of Recurrent Infections** Trimethoprim/ sulfamethoxazole Nitrofurantoin Trimethoprim

REVIEW QUESTIONS

ANTICHOLINERGIC DRUGS FOR OVERACTIVE BLADDER

Overactive bladder is characterized by: 1) urinary urgency; 2) urinary frequency; 3) nocturia; and 4) urge incontinence. Behavioural therapy is always encouraged as a first line treatment (scheduled voiding, timing fluid intake, Kegel exercise, avoiding caffeine). Studies have shown the current medical treatment for this disorder is just slightly higher than placebo effects (p. 121). This class of medications is aimed at blocking Muscarinic Subtype M3 Receptors in the bladder; however, these receptors are also included on the salivary glands, GI smooth muscle, eyes (iris sphincter, ciliary muscle, lacrimal gland). The action of these medications is to *block* M3 Receptors resulting in side effects such as: dry mouth, bladder relaxation (decreased pressure), constipation, mydriasis, blurred vision and dry eyes (p. 121). Also, if the drugs are non-selective for M3 receptors they can also influence M1 (salivary glands and CNS) and M2 (on the heart) receptors; this causes: dry mouth, confusion, hallucinations and tachycardia.

1. Make drug cards for Oxybutynin, Darifenacin and Solifenacin. What are common side effects with these medications? Are there any noted differences? What are common routes?
2. What are signs of antimuscarinic poisoning?
3. How would a nurse differentiate antimuscarinic poisoning from acute psychosis?
4. What is the antidote for muscarinic antagonist poisoning?

DRUGS TO TREAT URINARY RETENTION

1. Bethanechol is contraindicated for clients with PUD, urinary tract obstruction, intestinal obstruction, coronary insufficiency, hypotension, asthma and hyperthyroidism. Draw links between the pharmacodynamics of this medication and these conditions.
2. How does an overdose of this medication present clinically? What is the treatment for an overdose of bethanechol?

DRUG THERAPY FOR URINARY TRACT INFECTIONS

The majority of these medications are covered in the Anti-infective module in the study guide. The questions below focus on drugs not covered in detail in the Anti-infective module.

1. Nitrofurantoin is indicated for acute infections of the lower urinary tract. What colour does this medication turn the urine?
2. The following adverse effects are associated with the administration of Nitrofurantoin. Outline the potential assessment findings in a client experiencing these adverse effects due to drug therapy:

Adverse Effect	Assessment and/or Laboratory Findings:
Pulmonary reactions: acute and sub-acute	
Agranulocytosis	
Leukopenia	
Thrombocytopenia	
Megaloblastic anemia	
Peripheral Neuropathy	
Hepatotoxicity	

3. Ciprofloxacin poses a risk of phototoxicity. What are signs of this side effect and what are priority areas for client education?
4. Which type of bacterial infection is commonly associated with administration of ciprofloxacin?
5. Which drug levels can be elevated by ciprofloxacin?
6. The following should be administered at least 6 hours before or 2 hours after ciprofloxacin: aluminum or magnesium-containing antacids, iron salts, zinc salts, sucralfate, calcium supplements and milk or other dairy products. What is the rationale for this?
7. Trimethoprim/Sulfamethoxazole (Bactrim/Septra/Co-Trimoxazole) can cause varying adverse events. Name the most common.
8. Describe how the nurse can prevent cystalluria in clients taking trimethoprim/sulfamethoxazole.
9. In order to understand the full range of adverse effects of trimethoprim and sulfamethoxazole it is important to know each drug separately. Create a table outlining the adverse effects associated with 1) trimethoprim and 2) sulfamethoxazole.
10. What is Steven-Johnson's syndrome and which drug is it related to? What are the signs and symptoms of this condition?

Tips for answering exam questions related to these medications (Rosenjack Burchum et al., 2016):

- Ciprofloxacin and levofloxacin are the only fluoroquinolones approved for use in children
- Tendon damage is associated with fluoroquinolones (e.g., ciprofloxacin, levofloxacin, moxifloxacin)
- Moxifloxacin can cause QT prolongation
- Ciprofloxacin, norfloxacin and ofloxacin can increase warfarin levels
- Ciprofloxacin and ofloxacin can increase theophylline levels

PRACTICE QUESTIONS

Question 1
A client is receiving bethanechol to treat urinary retention. On assessment the client is salivating excessively, sweating, hypotensive and bradycardic. Which of the following nursing interventions is critical in this situation?

1. Administer physostigmine as per Health Care Provider's order
2. Administer atropine as per Health Care Provider's order and implement supportive measures
3. Discontinue the medication and implement supportive measures for the client
4. Call the Health Care Provider and prepare to administer a fluid bolus

Question 2
What is the colour of urine in a client receiving Nitrofurantoin therapy?

1. Bright red
2. Green tinged
3. Light brown
4. Straw-coloured

Question 3
A client is receiving Ciprofloxacin. What should the nurse teach the client regarding this medication?

1. To monitor the colour and consistency of their urine during drug therapy
2. To avoid prolonged exposure to sunlight and if outside to wear sunscreen and a hat
3. To assess for signs of renal impairment such as decreased urine output
4. To monitor to improvements in urinary frequency

Question 4
A client is receiving trimethoprim orally to treat a urinary tract infection. Which of the following clients would trimethoprim therapy absolutely contraindicated in?

1. Clients with a folate acid deficiency manifested as megaloblastic anemia
2. Clients with known hypokalemia
3. Clients with known kidney disease
4. Clients with urinary tract infections

Question 5
A client is experiencing cystalluria due to trimethoprim/sulfamethoxazole therapy. What should the nurse do to prevent this condition in future clients taking this therapy?

1. Teach the client to assess their urine output daily
2. Outline how to adhere to a low protein diet
3. Encourage the client to drink 6-8 glasses of water per day
4. Recommend that the client follow-up regularly with their Health Care Provider

Question 6
A client is receiving furosemide therapy. Which of the following adverse effects of this medication is the client at risk for? **(Select all that apply)**

1. Otoxicity
2. Hypokalemia
3. Hypotension
4. Hyperkalemia
5. Hyperuremia

Answers: Question 1(2), Question 2(3), Question 3 (2), Question 4(1), Question 5(3), Question 6 (1,2,3,5)

Study Strategy

This study guide differs from other resources because formal rationale is not provided for the answers. **You need to determine the appropriate rationale for the correct answers by accessing the information in the question that may have inhibited your ability to answer the question correctly**. It is helpful to ask the following questions:

- What is the question asking? What are key words in the question query?
- What information do I need to know to answer this question correctly?
- How did I select my answer?
- Why were the other answers incorrect?
- Was I missing a piece of content knowledge that inhibited how I answered the question? If so, what should I target in on and study?

Additional Strategies for Working with the Pharmacology Study Guide Modules

Content review is essential for being successful at answering NCLEX-RN® exam questions focusing on pharmacology. The following tips will help you to navigate the breath of this content and to organize your study notes. **Remember that you need to do the work of solid content review in order to be successful in understanding pharmacological concepts. Do not rely on practice questions to teach you what you need to know regarding medications for the NCLEX-RN®- practice questions are a tool for consolidating knowledge not a primary way to study.**

1. Complete the exercises in this study guide and make notes. This guide has been designed to direct you to important content for medication review. When creating the study guide I used an educator's lens to pull out the most important information in order ensure client safety with drug administration. For example, when review differing drugs I focused on critical information and essential education for each drug. The review questions are designed to bring this information forward.
2. Find ways to colour code or organize medications according to the bodily system or pathology they are used for. This will help you with recalling information. This guide uses a systems approach to help you organize the vast amount of pharmacological review in a way that will help you understand key concepts and pathologies.
3. Create case studies or unique ways to remember classes of medications. It is always wise to study pharmacology in the context of pathology. Use case studies specifically for content that is new to you or more difficult. Case studies should be memorable, contain client information that is easy to remember, focus on adverse effects of medications and key aspects of client education.

4. It is helpful to find patterns in names in drugs- such as suffixes that are common. Highlight the endings of common terms and find strategies to remember the main side effects of these classes of medications.
5. Client teaching is essential in medication administration. Ensure that you review your client education chapter in your Fundamentals of Nursing textbook (e.g. Potter and Perry). You need to remember that the use of basic teaching and learning principles paired with your knowledge of medications can help you to better exam questions.
6. When you use practice questions find consistent strategies for reviewing questions that you get incorrect. For example, the summary drug tables presented in each module of this guide provide a structure for organizing information. Create a blank table with the drug classes named for each system. Write information or content that is tested in each drug class as you move through your practice resources. Highlight the medication names you have seen in the practice questions on your summary table. Are there any patterns in the types of questions asked or the content tested? **Do be careful with this strategy- it is not a replacement for reviewing content.**

Conclusion

Strong pharmacological review will not only increase your chances of success on the NCLEX-RN® it will also strengthen your future nursing practice. The complexity of client care paired with the increase in co-morbidity and chronic disease management poses many challenges to pharmacological therapy. Nurses must be aware of potential drug-to-drug interactions, polypharmacy, and adverse events related to medications in order to keep their clients safe. I wish you all the best for your NCLEX-RN® exam and for your future nursing practice.

Best wishes,

Dr. Marnie Kramer-Kile

REFERENCES

Copstead, L.E & Banaski, J. (2013). *Pathophysiology* (5th ed). St. Louis: Elsevier.

Richards, J.S. (2013). Overview of herbal supplements. *Elite Continuing Education*, 46-72.

Rosenjack Burchum, J. & Rosenthal, L.D. (2016). *Lehne's pharmacology for nursing care* (9th edition). St. Louis: Elsevier.

Module 7

Anti-Infective Medications

TABLE OF CONTENTS

Tables and Figures

Introduction to the Transitioning to the NCLEX-RN® Pharmacology Guide: Anti-Infective Medications

The breadth and detail of the knowledge required of pharmacological concepts often overwhelms new graduates when they are beginning their exam preparation. The purpose of this pharmacology study guide is to help you work through the vast amount of pharmacological knowledge required for the NCLEX-RN® in a systematic and purposeful way. This guide organizes content using the current NCLEX-RN® Test Plan and provides specific strategies to address pharmacological areas of review which may challenge new graduates. **This is the seventh of twelve modules.** This is a working guide, so while key information will be presented and organized for review, it is up to you to do the detailed work of content review by answering the questions and exercises in each section. You can expect to see drugs described by their generic names on the exam. Due to the differences in drug trade names between the United States of America, Canada and other countries you should study drugs according to their generic names and develop strategies for remembering them.

This module is part of a comprehensive pharmacology study guide focusing on specific areas which may challenge NCLEX-RN® candidates. This includes drug-to-drug interactions, specific adverse reactions due to drug therapy and the potential reactions associated with herbal therapy and conventional medications. The content will be focused on a systems approach and will direct you towards important information within each drug class.

Structure of the Module

This module begins with an overview of the differing drug classes of Anti-Infective Therapy. Additional areas for review that are specialized or affect multiple systems will also be highlighted:

1. Review questions and selected exercises will be constructed for each drug class to help pull out key concepts such as adverse events/side effects, specific client teaching and drug to drug interactions.
2. A summary chart of the drug classes in each system or theme will be provided for you to use alongside practice questions. As you move through practice questions, check off the specific medications you come across and if you require further review in each area. It is also helpful to make your own drug cards for specific medications. Keep the drug cards simple. Identify the drug class, the mechanism of action, two relevant (i.e., life threatening) or unique adverse effects that require monitoring and provide an outline for client teaching or specific nursing interventions for the medication.

Advice for Studying Pharmacological Content for the NCLEX-RN®

Always start with areas you are NOT familiar with. For example, if you spent the majority of your time as a final practicum student/or nurse on a cardiology unit do not start in the Vascular and Cardiac Medications Module. It is common for students/graduates to move to areas of comfort when they are studying because it decreases their anxiety. However, your efforts should be targeted on what you don't know. Each Module in this guide has a summary table of drugs for each system. Highlight the drug classes that you are not familiar with and make it your priority to work through them. Do not spend time making drug cards for medications you already know. For example, most students are confident with furosemide administration and can critically think through concepts associated with the drug. Therefore, time does not need to be spent studying this medication. Only make drug cards for medications that are new to you. The review questions in this guide will direct you towards more detailed information of the medications that you are familiar with and focus on potential areas where exam questions may be asked.

This guide is set up using a **systems approach** for the following reasons: 1) most pharmacology textbooks use this approach to structure content so it will be easier to find the information you need to answer the review questions; 2) using a systems approach allows you to find commonalties in the side effects of drugs influencing a specific system, so you will see patterns arising as you work through this guide; and 3) a systems approach allows for the creation of overall drug summary tables, which will be included in each module of the guide and will provide you with a general sense of the medications you need to cover.

The following resources will aid you in answering questions posed in this guide. This includes:

1. **A pharmacology textbook.** This resource will contain more detailed information pertaining to drug classes and outline general nursing considerations for therapy. I have referenced a pharmacology textbook throughout the writing of this guide.
2. **A drug guide**. These are the guides commonly used for your clinical practice. These resources contain alphabetized drug information. Most importantly, they outline specific pharmacokinetic and pharmacodynamics properties of drugs. You will find information related to drug excretion, protein binding, and therapeutic index in these guides.
3. **An online drug repository** for more detailed information that may not be found in the two resources above. Sometimes it is difficult to find therapeutic index and protein binding for a drug. I have found the following website helpful for this: http://www.drugbank.ca/drugs

Module 7: Anti-Infective Medications

This module covers anti-infective medications and medications for the treatment of HIV infections. Key drug classes will be covered and review questions will be posed. This module is divided into three separate parts: 1) Anti-infective medications; 2) Antiviral Therapy (Non-HIV related, and 3) HIV Antiviral therapy. It is essential that you understand how the body reacts to both bacterial and viral infections. Antibiotic and antiviral therapy has many adverse effects and drug-to-drug interactions. This module focuses primarily on these concepts. There are parts of this module that you may find tedious, particularly the in-depth content on HIV Antiretroviral medication. However, in my exploration of various NCLEX-RN® resources questions related to these medications often focus on in-depth concepts. It is important that you work through the exercises provided and ensure that you understand the underlying pathophysiology involved in this therapy.

Part 1: Anti-Infective Medications

The first table highlights common classes of anti-infective medications. The review questions will focus on Anti-Fungal Drugs and Drugs for Tuberculosis only. The remaining drug classes will be presented in a summary table, followed by a summary exercise to help you pull out the most important concepts coming forward in the content.

Terminology/Concepts to Review for Anti-Infective Medications

It is important that you understand the following terminology and concepts that apply to the administration of anti-infective therapy:

- Gram –ve vs. Gram +ve bacteria and how this influences the selection of anti-infective therapy
- Selective toxicity
- Broad vs. narrow spectrum antibiotics
- Antibiotic resistance (role of NDM-1 gene in bacterial resistance); ways to delay antibiotic resistance
- Minimum inhibitory concentration (MIC) of antibiotics
- Minimum bactericidal concentration (MBC)
- Bactericidal vs. bacteriostatic properties of antibiotics/anti-infective medications
- Recommended treatment for a Clostridium difficile infection
- Signs of C-Difficile Associated Diarrhea (CDAD)

Table 7.1 Summary of Anti-Infective Medications

Penicillins:	**Cephalosporins**	**Tetracyclines**	**Aminoglycosides**
Amoxicillin	Cefaclor	Demeclocycline	Gentamicin
Amoxicillin/	Cefadroxil	Doxycycline	Tobramycin
clavulanate	Cefazolin	Minocycline	Amikacin
Ampicillin	Cefdinir	Tetracycline	Kanamycin
Ampicillin/sulbactam	Cefditoren		Neomycin
Dicloxacillin	Cefepime	**Macrolides**	Paromomycin
Nafcillin	Cefixime	Erythromycin	Streptomycin
Oxacillin	Cefotaxime	Clarithromycin	
Penicillin G	Cefotetan	Azithromycin	
Penicillin V	Cefoxitin		**Drugs for**
Piperacillin	Cefpodoxime	**Other**	**Tuberculosis**
Piperacillin	Cefprozil	**Bacteriostatic**	Isoniazid
Piperacillin/	Ceftaroline	**Inhibitors of**	Rifampin
tazobactam	Ceftazidime	**Protein Synthesis**	Rifapentine
Ticarcillin/clavulanate	Ceftibuten	Clindamycin	Ribabutin
	Cefriaxone	Linezolid	Pyrazinamide
	Cefurosime	Telithromycin	Ethambutol
Drugs for Leprosy	Cephalexin	Dalfopristin/	Bedaquiline
(Hansen's Disease)		Quinupristin	
Rifampin	**Sulfonamides**	Chloramphenicol	**Antifungal**
Dapsone	Sulfadiazine	Tigecycline	**Agents**
Ofloxacin	Sulfamethoxazole	Retapamulin	Amphotericin B
Minocycline	Sulfisoxazole	Mupirocin	Itraconazole
			Fluconazole
Fluoroquinolones			Ketoconazole
Ciprofloxin			Flucoytosine
			Caspofungin

ANTIFUNGAL AGENTS

1. Amphotericin B is given for systemic mycoses via IV and intrathecal routes. It has serious adverse effects. Outline the nursing interventions required to both assess for and treat potential adverse effects associated with this medication:

Adverse Effect	**Nursing Assessments and/or Interventions**
Fever, chills, rigors, nausea, headache	
Nephrotoxicity	
Hypokalemia	
Hematologic effects: normocytic, normochromic anemia	

2. Itraconazole can cause liver injury and cardiac suppression. What are signs that these side effects are occurring?

3. Itraconazole can raise levels of pimoide, quinidine, dofetilide and cisapride—what is the potential lethal effect from toxic levels of these medications?
4. Itraconazole levels can be decreased by any medications that raise gastric pH. Identify potential medication classes that may influence the absorption of itraconazole. What should the nurse teach clients using itraconazole when taking these agents?
5. Make drug cards for the remaining antifungal agents on the list above. Focus in on client teaching and potential adverse events.
6. Some of the "azole" drugs can cause excessive and fatal adverse effects by raising the levels of other drugs. Complete the following table to review these medications:

Drug Level Raised by Azole Drug	Class of Drug	Consequence of Excessive Level	Nursing Assessment
Pimozide			
Dofetilide			
Quinidine			
Cisapride			
Warfarin			
Sulfonylureas			
Phenytoin			
Cyclosporine			
Tacrolimus			
Lovastatin			
Simvastatin			
Fentanyl			
Calcium Channel Blockers			
Eletriptan			

DRUGS FOR TUBERCULOSIS

Promoting adherence and multi-drug therapy are major focuses for client education. Adherence can be increased by using directly observed therapy (DOT). Treatment is considered successful if there is: 1) reduction in fever, malaise, anorexia, cough and other clinical manifestations (2 weeks), 2) radiographic evidence of improvement (3 months), and 3) absence of *M. tuberculosis* in sputum (3-6 months).

1. Begin by making drug cards for isoniazid, rifampin, pyrazinamide and ethambutol. Each drug has specific abnormal adverse effects; ensure you are familiar with them.

2. How does drug therapy for tuberculosis differ in clients that are HIV +ve? What are the potential consequences of rifampin NOT being administered to these clients?
3. What is the treatment if infecting organisms are not resistant to isoniazid or rifampin? Include the induction and continuance phases of treatment.
4. How is isoniazide or rifampin-resistant tuberculosis treated?

Study Strategy

Refer to the Antibiotic Summary Table (7.2) below to review the major drug classes. Use the drug list at the start of this chapter to organize your approach to this content area. Make drug cards for each anti-infective listed. It is also helpful to keep track of the themes in practice questions regarding this content. Create a blank table with the drug classes listed and keep notes on each class as you work through practice questions.

Table 7.2 Summary of Common Anti-Infective Drug Classes

Drug Class	Action	Bacteria	Broad/ Narrow Spectrum	Adverse Effects	Nursing Considerations
Penicillins	**Bactericidal** Weakens cell wall; kills bacteria by interfering with its ability to synthesize the cell wall, the bacteria lengthen but cannot divide, eventually the weak cell wall ruptures.	Gram +ve Gram –ve (only certain penicillins will work)	Broad Narrow	• Severe anaphylaxis in some pts • Sodium loading can occur in high doses of ticarcillin/clavulanate or sodium penicillin G • Potassium overloading in potassium penicillin G • Pencillins can inactivate aminoglycosides	• Drug resistance may occur • Monitor kidney function, assess for history of allergic reactions, monitor for allergic reactions, monitor for pseudomembranous colitis • Assess for history of severe allergic reactions to penicillins, cephalosporins or carbapenems • Oral penicillin is taken with a full glass of water 1 hour before meals or 2 hours after • Always teach the client to take full prescribed treatment • Treat anaphylaxis with epinephrine (sc, IM, or IV) and respiratory support

Cephalosporins *often indicated for pts who cannot tolerate penicillin* **Review the 5 generations of these drugs** 5-10% chance that if you react to penicillin you will react to these drugs	**Bactericidal** Weaken cell wall, causing lysis and bacteria's death. Used in pts who cannot tolerate penicillin. 4 generations of this class of drugs	Gram +ve Gram –ve (depends on generation of drug used)		• Bleeding—cefotetan and ceftriazone by reducing prothrombin levels via interference with Vit K metabolism (stop drug and tx with Vit K) • May cause antibuse like reactions with ETOH (cefazolin, cefotetan). • Pseudomembranous colitis • Hemolytic anemia • IV Ceftriaxone & IV Calcium given together can cause precipitates in the body and death!	• Assess for history of bleeding disorders as these drugs may interfere with Vit. K metabolism • Assess liver function as it also plays a role in Vit. K production • Teach pts to avoid alcohol • Assess renal function (excreted through kidneys) • Administered IM or IV—poor absorption in GI tract • IM injections of these drugs are painful—warn client • Do not give cefditoren tablets to clients with milk allergies—the drug contains a milk protein
Tetracyclines Treatment of: Infectious disease Acne Peptic Ulcer Disease Periodontal Disease	Bacteriostatic Inhibits bacterial protein synthesis.	Gram +ve Gram -ve	Broad	• May cause photosensitivity • Binds with Ca and iron should not be taken with milk or iron supplements (decreases absorption) • GI Irritation • Superinfection • Hepatotoxicity • Renal toxicity • Photosensitivity	• Milk and cheese result in decreased drug level • Decreased efficacy when used with oral contraceptives • Binds with developing teeth, if taken by children 4 months to 8 years of age teeth will be permanently stained. Not recommended for children less than 8 years. • Can increase digoxin levels through increasing absorption in the GI tract • Increases INR levels by altering Vit K producing flora in the gut

Macrolides (erythromycin)	**Bacteriostatic** Inhibits bacterial protein synthesis. Indicated for respiratory, GI tract, skin and soft tissue infections, otitis media, gonorrhea, non-gonococcal urethritis, *H. pylori*	Gram +ve Gram -ve	Broad	• Toxic effects to the liver (hepatotoxicity—must monitor liver enzymes; do not give to a pt. with liver disease) • QT prolongation and sudden cardiac death • Gastrointestinal effects	• Need to monitor drug levels • Assess for hx of heart disease (may worsen symptoms) • Assess liver enzymes regularly • Look for rashes or other signs of hypersensitivity (Stevens-Johnson Syndrome) • May decrease warfarin metabolism and excretion; monitor INR more frequently • Can also increase theophylline & carbamazepine levels • Do not take with fruit juices • Always finish full medication regime
Aminoglycosides (gentamycin) Samples for **peak** levels should be taken 30 min after giving IM injection or after completing a 30 min IV infusion Samples for **trough** levels depends on dosing schedule:	**Bactericidal** Disrupt protein synthesis and causes synthesis of abnormal proteins. Reserved for serious systemic infections	Gram -ve	Narrow	• **Ototoxicity** (Hearing loss) • **Nephrotoxicity** (increases with high trough levels) • Suprainfection • May cause neuromuscular blockade (not being able to move) in patients receiving anesthetics.	• Give via IV (poor absorption in GI tract) • Assess client for history of previous allergic reaction • Do baseline audiometry, renal function, vestibular function • May cause greater muscle weakness in pts with neuromuscular disease • Promote fluid intake • Frequently combined with penicillins, cephalosporins and vancomycin for a greater kill rate of bacteria (however, concurrent therapy increases risk of nephrotoxicity) • Monitor serum drug levels

Divided doses: taken just before next dose **Single daily doses**: 1 hour before next dose *The lab value should be close to 0					
Fluoroquinolones (e.g., ciprofloxacin)	**Bactericidal** Affects DNA synthesis by inhibiting two bacterial enzymes: DNA gyrase and topoisomerase IV Not first line drugs but used as alternatives to other antibiotics Respiratory, GI, gynecological tracts, some skin and soft tissue infections	Gram –ve Gram +ve	Narrow and Broad spectrum	• Leucopenia, dysrhythmias, liver failure, CNS disturbances • Dysrhythmias and liver failure	• Increase fluid intake to decrease crystalluria (monitor i & o) • May cause light-headedness (pt should not drive) • Do not take concurrently with multi-vitamins or mineral supplements (can reduce absorption of drug by 90%) • Monitor CBC & diff. • Use cautiously in children • Report signs of tendon inflammation

Sulfonamides (e.g., trimethoprim-sulfamethoxazole known as Bactrim, Novo-Trimel, Septra)	Generally safe drugs but some side effects can be serious. Classified by their absorption and excretion characteristics	Gram +ve Gram -ve	Broad	• Fatal blood abnormalities: aplastic anemia, hemolytic anemia, agranulocytosis. • Crystals in the urine (renal damage). • Stevens-Johnson syndrome • Kernicterus in Newborns	• Assess for anemia and other hematological disorder • Avoid exposure to direct sunlight, take with full glass of water, increase fluid intake (may cause crystals to form in the urine and block the kidney), monitor kidney function, report side effects immediately • Advise clients to consume 8-10 glasses of water per day (require daily urine outflow of 1200mL per day)
Miscellaneous Antibacterials: **Clindamycin** Indications are limited due to risk of CDAD Used for gas gangrene infections	Drug of choice for oral infections.	Gram +ve Gram -ve	Broad	• Do not give in pts with history of inflammatory bowel disease, regional enteritis • Associated with pseudomembranous colitis and c-difficile associated diarrhea (CDAD)	• Assess for pseudomembranous colitis and CDAD • Assess for hypersensitivity • Look for: diarrhea, rashes, difficulty breathing, itching and difficulty swallowing

Vancomycin	Reserved for severe infections Used after bacteria have become resistant to other antibiotics Used to treat MRSA Inhibits cell wall synthesis	Gram -ve	Narrow	• Red man syndrome: hypotension, flushing and red rash on face and upper body • Super-infection • Nephrotoxicity leading to anemia • Renal failure • Thrombophlebitis	• Renal function, urine output (reduce doses in renal impairment) • Assess hearing function • Assess for hypersensitivity reactions • Assess for Red man syndrome

Source: Rosenjack Burchum, J. & Rosenthal, L.D. (2016). Lehne's pharmacology for nursing care (9th ed.). St. Louis: Elsevier.

ADDITIONAL MEDICATIONS: ANTHELMINTICS (FOR PARASITIC WORMS)

Helminthic are parasitic worms. Typically most infections are asymptomatic and can occur inside or outside of the intestines. Treatment of helminths is not always indicated because most parasitic worms do not reproduce in the body. Health promotion, particularly in areas where worm infestations are common, is the best measure for prevention. These medications have very few side effects- with the majority being related to gastrointestinal upset (e.g. diarrhea, nausea, stomach pain, cramps). One medication, diethylcarbamazine can have indirect effects that result from the death of the worms- which can include rashes, intense itching, encephalitis, fever, tachycardia, lymphadenitis, leukocytosis and proteinuria- these symptoms are transient and just last a few days. Glucocorticoids can be given pre-treatment to minimize this response (Rosenjack Burchum, 2016, p.1185). Table 7.3 below contains a summary of these medications and types of infections they treat.

Table 7.3 Medications Given for Helminthic Infections

Worm Class	Common Name	Drug of Choice
Nematodes (roundworms) Intestinal	Giant roundworm Pinworm Hookworm Whipworm Threadworm	Albendzole or mebendazole or ivermectin Albendzole or mebendazole or pyrantel pamoate Albendzole or mebendazole or pyrantel pamoate Albendazole Ivermectin
Nematodes (roundworms) Extra-intestinal	Pork roundworm Filariae	Albendazole (although not FDA approved for this indication) Diethylcarbamazine, Ivermectin
Cestodes (tapeworms)	Beef tapeworm Pork tapeworm Fish tapeworm	Praziquantel (for all three)
Trematodes (flukes)	Blood fluke Intestinal fluke Lung fluke Liver flukes	Praziquantel Praziquantel Praziquantel Triclabendazole Praziquantel or albendazole

Source: Rosenjack Burchum, J. & Rosenthal, L.D. (2016). Lehne's pharmacology for nursing care (9th edition). St. Louis: Elsevier. p.1183

ADDITIONAL MEDICATIONS: ANTIMALARIAL AGENTS

Plasmodium will reside in the liver or erythrocytes. In order for symptoms of malaria to be cured the plasmodium must be eradicated in the erythrocytes. However, because the parasites also reside in the liver relapse can occur (with Plasmodium vivax infections)(p.1194). Study medications for the prophylaxis and treatment of malaria.

1. What are the two principal forms of malaria?
2. Which parasite is drug resistance the most common with? *Plasmodium flaiparum or Plasmodium vivax?*
3. Describe the mechanism of action, use and potential side effects of chloroquine. What is chloroquine resistance in the context of malaria?
4. Is primaquine more useful for erythrocytic or hepatic forms of malaria? What is the most serious adverse event associated with this drug?
5. How does quinine kill the malaria parasite? What is cinchonism and what are its symptoms?
6. Quinidine gluconate is the only drug approved for parenteral therapy of malaria. What drug should be given with quinine to enhance antiplasmodial effects? What are two serious adverse events associated with the IV administration of quinidine gluconate?
7. Mefloquine can prolong the QT interval and cause dysrhythmias. Which clients would be at an increased risk of this side effect and how would the nurse assess for a prolonged QT interval?

ADDITIONAL MEDICATIONS: ANTPROTOZOAL DRUGS MISCELLANEOUS AGENTS

The central focus in this section will be on the administration of metronidazole because it is one of the most common medications given. For your reference, other drugs for protozoal infections include: iodoquinol, tinidazole, benznidazole, nitazoxanide, pentamidine, suramin, melarsoprol, eflornithine, nifurtimox, pyrimethamine, sodium stibogluconate, miltefosine, and amphotericin B.

1. Metronidazole is the drug of choice for treating which type of infections?
2. Why is alcohol avoided for clients taking metronidazole?
3. Which serious hypersensitivity reaction is linked to metronidazole?
4. What are less serious, but notable, side effects which would not require termination of treatment?

Areas not covered in this section include: ectoparasites (e.g. lice, scabies, mites). It may be helpful to create a care plan for a client with a lice infection, especially within a pediatric context. Outline specific client teaching regarding any of the side effects of this treatment.

PRACTICE QUESTIONS

Question 1

Which of the following cardiac abnormalities would alert the nurse to a potentially life-threatening adverse effect of Erythromycin therapy?

1.

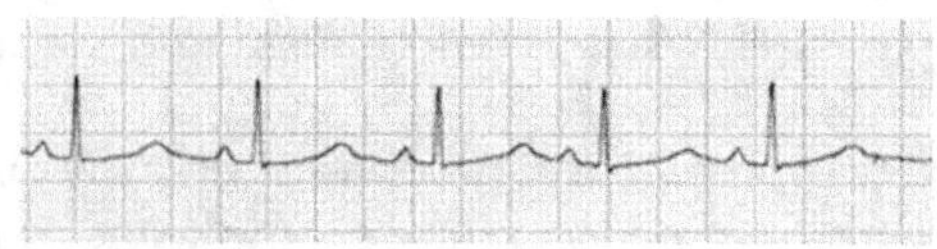

3.

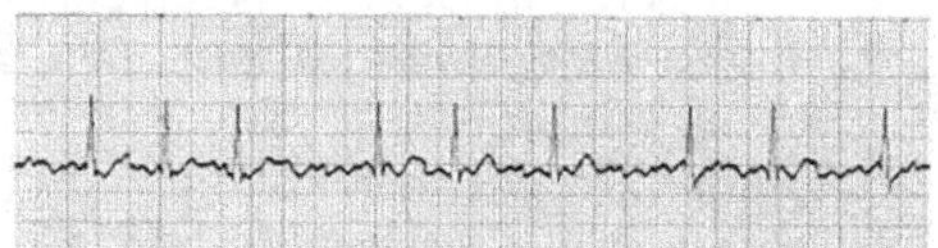

2.

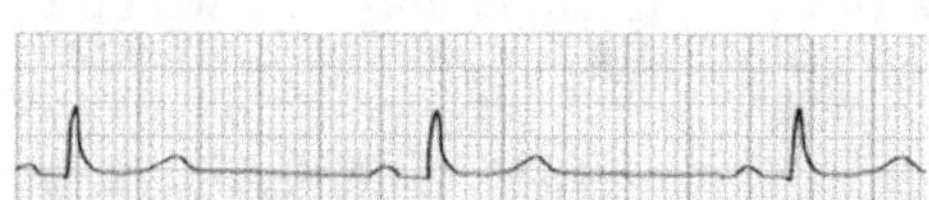

4.

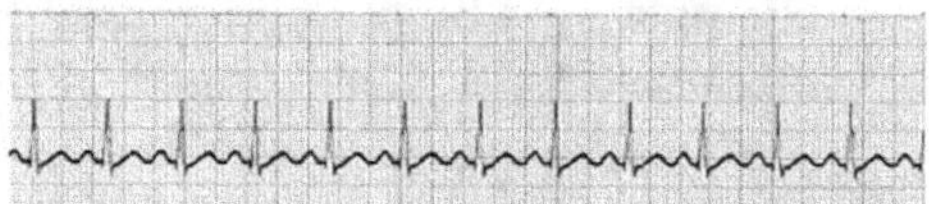

Question 2

A client with a history of chronic alcoholism requires antibiotic therapy. Which of the following medications would not be an appropriate choice due to their ability to cause a disulfiram-like reaction when combined with alcohol?

1. Cefaclor and cefazolin
2. Cefazolin and cefotetan
3. Erythromycin and penicillin G
4. Vancomycin and cefazolin

Question 3

A client is receiving gentamicin 5mg/kg IV daily at 0800h. The Health Care Provider has ordered a peak level to be drawn. If the infusion was started exactly at 0800h what time would the peak level be due?

1. 0730h
2. 0900h
3. 0830h
4. 1000h

Question 4

A client is receiving trimethoprim-sulfamethoxazole orally. Which of the following nursing interventions should the nurse focus on for a client receiving this drug therapy? **(Select all that apply)**

1. Assess if the client has a folic acid deficiency
2. Encourage the client to drink 8-10 glass of water per day
3. Check daily Creatinine and BUN levels
4. Instruct client to report any hearing loss
5. Teach the client to perform daily weights

Question 5

A client is receiving oral cefditoren therapy. The nurse is exploring food related allergies prior to administering this medication. Which of the following food allergies would contraindicate the administration of this medication?

1. Eggs
2. Shellfish
3. Milk, yogurt, cheese
4. Peanuts

Answers: Question 1(1), Question 2(2), Question 3 (3), Question 4(1,2,3), Question 5(3)

Study Strategy

This study guide differs from other resources because formal rationale is not provided for the answers. **You need to determine the appropriate rationale for the correct answers by accessing the information in the question that may have inhibited your ability to answer the question correctly.** It is helpful to ask the following questions:

- What is the question asking? What are key words in the question query?
- What information do I need to know to answer this question correctly?
- How did I select my answer?
- Why were the other answers incorrect?
- Was I missing a piece of content knowledge that inhibited how I answered the question? If so, what should I target in on and study?

Part Two: Anti-Viral Agents

Table 7.4 Anti-Viral Agents

Systemic Drugs for Herpes Simplex Viruses & Varicella-Zoster Virus Acyclovir Valacyclovir Famciclovir Foscarnet **Topical Drugs for Herpes Simplex Viruses & Varicella-Zoster Virus** Vidarabine Penciclovir Trifluidine Docosanol Ganciclovir	**Drugs for Hepatitis C** Interferon Alfa Ribavirin Boceprevir Telaprevir **Drugs for Hepatitis B** Interferon Alfa Nucleoside Analogs
Drugs for Cytomegalovirus Infection Ganciclovir Valganciclovir Cidofovir Foscarnet	**Drugs for Influenza** Oseltamivir Zanamivir **Drugs for Respiratory Syncytial Virus Infection** Ribavirin Palivizumab

REVIEW QUESTIONS

SYSTEMIC & TOPICAL DRUGS FOR HERPES SIMPLEX VIRUSES & VARICELLA-ZOSTER VIRUS

1. What are the therapeutic uses for Acyclovir? Why are clients on dialysis at risk for severe neurotoxicity when taking this medication?
2. Does Acyclovir cure herpes simplex genitalis?
3. Why is Valacyclovir indicated primarily for immunocompetent clients? What side effect can occur in clients who are immunocompromised?
4. Outline a teaching plan for a client who is using topical creams for Herpes Labialis (penciclovir cream, docosanol cream)

DRUGS FOR CYTOMEGALOVIRUS INFECTION

1. Review the transmission of CMV infections and where they occur in the body. Why is this type of infection severe in immunocompromised or pregnant clients?

2. Ganciclovir is used for the prevention and treatment of CMV infections in immunocompromised hosts. What the two severe side effects related to this medication? How would the nurse assess for these side effects?
3. What are the effects of ganciclovir on the reproductive system on both males and females?
4. Why should the nurse handle valganciclovir powder and tablets carefully? What can they cause if they contact the skin of the nurse?
5. Foscarnet can cause electrolyte depletion. What are common electrolytes influenced by this medication?

DRUGS FOR HEPATITIS

Hepatitis can be caused by six different hepatitis viruses (A, B, C, D, E, and G)—all of these viruses cause acute hepatitis but only B, C and D cause chronic hepatitis (Rosenjack Burchum et al., 2016, p. 1112). Hepatitis C and B will be the main focus of this section.

Hepatitis C

1. Interferon Alfa (Inferferon alfa-2b and interferon alfacon-1) are used for Chronic Hepatitis C. Identify the most common adverse effects associated with this therapy. What is the route used for medication administration?
2. Ribavirin is given orally and combined with SC peginterferon alfa—Ribavirin can cause hemolytic anemia. Outline the assessment findings in a client experiencing hemolytic anemia.
3. Boceprevir is a protease inhibitor. How does this class of medication work in the cell? Boceprevir will increase the levels of drugs and can alter other drug levels. There are too many drug-to-drug interactions to count with this medication, so keep this in mind as a primary concept when answering questions regarding this medication.
4. Telaprevir is also a protease inhibitor that must be combined with peginterferon alfa and ribavirin for therapy. It also causes anemia and one other potentially fatal hypersensitivy reaction. What is this condition called?

Hepatitis B (HBV)

**Interferon Alfa as identified above is also used to treat chronic hepatitis B*

1. Lamivudine is used for both HBV and HIV infections. What are 3 rare but dangerous adverse effects of this medication?
2. Why should HIV infection be ruled out in clients with HBV prior to administering Adefovir?

DRUGS FOR INFLUENZA

1. Oseltamivir (Tamiflu) must be started no later than 2 days after symptom onset. Why is this? What are adverse effects of this medication?
2. A client is getting the flu shot (Live Influenza Vaccine). How does this influence the administration of oseltamivir?
3. How is Zanamivir administered? How should the nurse teach the client to take this medication?

DRUGS FOR RESPIRATORY SYNCYTIAL VIRUS INFECTION

1. Ribavirin is a broad-spectrum antiviral drug in aerosol and oral preparations. It is used for severe viral pneumonia caused by RSV. Although its adverse effects are limited, it does pose a risk to infants on mechanical ventilation. Why?
2. Pavlivizumab is used to prevent RSV in infants and young children with chronic lung disease. It can cause hypersensitivity reactions. How would a hypersensitivity reaction be managed?

Part 3: Antiviral Agents for HIV-Related Infections

It is important for you to review the Replication Cycle of the Human Immunodeficiency Virus. This is key in understanding the mechanism of actions of these medications. The following questions will help to direct you to important content:

1. What are the 10 steps in the Replication Cycle of HIV? Draw out the cell and the steps involved.
2. What are signs of acute retroviral syndrome?
3. Review the transmission of HIV.
4. What is the difference between HIV-1 and HIV-2 infections? How does this influence drug treatment?

One of the most challenging aspects of learning about antiretroviral drugs is understanding how they work in the virial replication cycle and the complexity of adverse effects and drug-to-drug interactions. Many of the adverse reactions occur with increased dosing of the medications. The review questions in this section will focus in on these higher level concepts. It is helpful for you to create drug cards for at least 1-2 medications in each of the drug classes listed in the table above.

The following link takes you to a helpful online module for HIV treatment and pharmacology

http://i-base.info/course-materials-introduction-course/

Table 7.5 Antiviral Agents for HIV-Related Infections

Nucleoside/Nucleotide reverse Transcriptase Inhibitors	**Non-Nucleoside Reverse Transcriptase Inhibitors**	**Protease Inhibitors**
Abacavir Zidovudine Didanosine Tenofovir Emtricitabine Stavudine Lamivudine	Delavirdine Efavirenz Etravirine Nevirapine Rilpivirine	Atazanavir Tipranavir Darunavir Saquinavir Fosamprenavir Rionavir Indinavir Nelfinavir Lopinavir/Ritonavir
Antiviral Agents for HIV Infection Retrieved from: http://i-base.info/course-materials-introduction-course/		
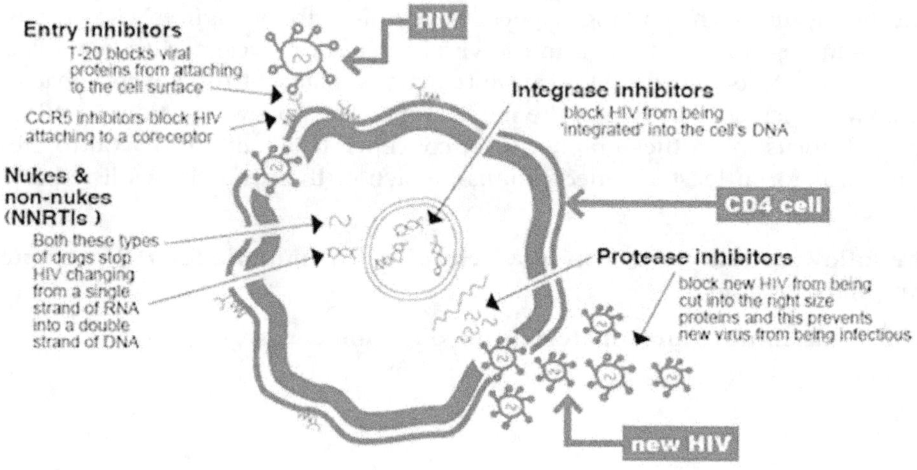 **HIV Fusion Inhibitor** Enfuvirtide	**CCR5 Antagonist** Maraviroc	**Integrase Strand Transfer Inhibitor** Raltegravir

REVIEW QUESTIONS

1. Zidovudine (Abbreviations are ZDV and AZT—for azidothymidine, its original name) was the first NRTI available. It is employed in combination with other antiretroviral drugs. What are the two major side effects of this medication?
2. Why would folic acid and vitamin B12 deficiencies make the side effects of Zidovudine worse?

3. Lactic acidosis with hepatomegaly and myopathy are also associated with Zidovudine. Outline how the nurse would assess for these two complications.
4. Drugs that cause any type of myelosuppressive, nephrotoxic or directly toxic to circulating blood cells can increase the risk of Zidovudine-induced hematologic toxicity (Rosenjack Burchum et al., 2016, p.1129). Identify two drugs that may potentiate this effect when administered with Zidovudine.
5. What happens if therapy with Emtricitabine, Tenofovir or Lamivudine is withdrawn in a client who has HIV and Hepatitis B?

The following Table 7.6 highlights common adverse effects of these medications and outlines some of the more specific and unique adverse effects of these medications. Find a strategy for remembering these key points regarding this class of medications.

Table 7.6 Adverse Effects of NNRI's

Drug Name	Abacavir (ABC)	Didanosine (ddl)	Emtricitabine (FTC)	Lamivudine (3TC)	Stavudine (d4T)	Tenofovir (TDF)	Zidovudine (ZDV)
Common Adverse Effects shared with other NRTI's	Lactic Acidosis Increased risk of MI	Lactic Acidosis Increased risk of MI Insulin Resistance DM Pancreatitis	Lactic Acidosis	Lactic Acidosis	Lactic Acidosis Pancreatitis Insulin Resistance DM Hyperlipidemia Lipoatrophy	Lactic Acidosis	Lactic Acidosis Hyperlipidemia Lipoatrophy Insulin Resistance DM
Specific to the Drug	Hypersensitivity Reactions	Peripheral Neuropathy Retinal Changes	Hyperpigmentation of palms & soles	Minimal Toxicity	Hyperlipidemia Rapidly progressive neuromuscular weakness (rare)	Renal insufficiency Osteomalacia	Bone marrow suppression Myopathy Nail pigmentation

6. Understanding Drug-to-Drug Interactions with NRTI therapy:
   In studying the wide range of various drug-to-drug interactions with this class of medications it is important to focus on the potential reactions:
   a. Alcohol will cause toxicity of most of these medications and increase the risk of the client developing pancreatitis
   b. Some drugs will elevate the levels of NTRI drugs
   c. Some NTRI drugs will decrease the levels of other drugs
   d. NTRI therapy given with other drugs will sometimes increase the risk for hepatotoxicity, neuropathy or depress the immune response
7. Complete the following table below in order to gain an understanding of some of the more prominent drug-to-drug interactions:

NRTI Drug	Drug-to-Drug Interactions
Abacavir	
Didanosine	
Emtricitabine	
Lamivudine	
Stavudine	
Tenofovir	
Zidovudine	

NON-NUCLEOSIDE REVERSE TRANSCRIPTASE INHIBITORS (NNRTI's)

1. How do NNTRIs differ from NTRIs in their structure and mechanism of action?
2. Efavirenz is the only NNTRI recommended as first line therapy for HIV infection. What are noted adverse effects of this medication?
3. Women taking Efavirenz cannot get pregnant- it is recommended that they use both a hormonal contraceptive and barrier contraception. Why? (hint: Efavirenz has drug-to-drug interactions with oral contraceptives—what are they?)

PROTEASE INHIBITORS

This class of medication when combined with NRTIs can reduce viral load to a level that is undetectable. It is helpful to focus on the group properties of these medications in the context of adverse effects. These drugs **end with "vir"** and include: Atazanavir, Darunavir Fosamprenavir, Indinavir, Lopinavir/Ritonavir, Nelfinavir, Rionavir, Saquinavir and Tipranavir.

Complete the following summary table regarding the most common adverse effects of protease inhibitors:

Adverse Effects	Identification and Management of Side Effect
Hyperglycemia/Diabetes	
Fat Redistribution	
Hyperlipidemia	
Increased bleeding in clients with Hemophilia	
Reduced Bone Marrow Density	
Elevation of Serum Transaminases	

Integrative Therapy Caution

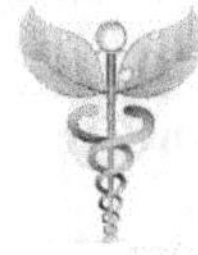

Herbal Medication: Garlic

Use of garlic supplements with HIV Protease Inhibitors (PI) may decrease PI drug levels. Garlic also influences blood clotting and blood sugar levels. Has the potential to increase bleeding in clients taking ASA, warfarin, or clopidogrel (Richards, 2013).

INTEGRASE STRAND TRANSFER INHIBITOR

1. Raltegravir is active against HIV strains resistant to other drugs and is indicated for combined use with other antiretroviral agents to treat adults with HIV-1. Which other NRTI's is this medication typically combined with for first-line therapy of HIV-1?
2. What are potential drug-to-drug interactions associated with raltegravir?

CCR5 ANTAGONIST

1. How does Maraviroc work? Why is CCR5 an essential aspect for HIV replication?
2. Levels of this drug are raised by several protease inhibitors. Which drugs **lower** the levels of this medication?

HIV FUSION INHIBITOR

1. What is the mechanism of action of Enfuvirtide?
2. This drug is given twice daily via sc injection. Injection-site reactions occur in nearly all clients. What are these reactions?
3. Enfurvirtide also increases the risk of pneumonia. What would the nurse teach the client regarding the signs and symptoms of this side effect?

PRACTICE QUESTIONS

Question 1
Which of the following medications is most likely to cause this adverse effect with administration?

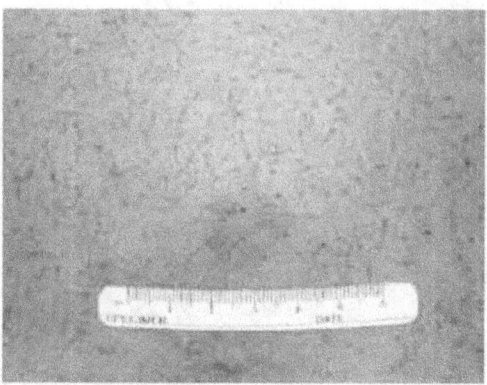

Retrieved from: http://www.thebody.com/multidrug/images/truth_reactions.jpg

1. Maraviroc 150 mg po twice daily
2. Enfuvirtide 90mg sc twice daily
3. Zidovudine 300mg IV twice daily
4. Rilivirine 25mg po once daily

Question 2
A client taking NRTI and Protease Inhibitor therapy viral load is now undetectable. What is a priority area for client education in order to promote health and safety?

1. Ensure the client understands they need to keep taking the medication
2. Educate that although the HIV RNA is undetectable that they are still infectious
3. Advise the client that they will need to stop and then re-continue therapy once their viral load is detectable again
4. Teach the client to contact the nurse if they have any signs of infection

Question 3
A female client is taking Nevirapine as part of their NNRTI drug therapy. Which of the following herbal medications is contraindicated with use of this medication?

1. Kava kava
2. Valerian root
3. St. John's wort
4. Melatonin

Question 4
A client has been taking Lopinavir/ Ritonavir for the past month. Which of the following signs and symptoms associated with this drug therapy should the client report to the nurse immediately? **(Select all that apply).**

1. Polyuria
2. Polydipsia
3. Polyphagia
4. Pruritus
5. Premature ventricular contractions

Question 5
A client is taking maraviroc daily for the past two months. Which of the following symptoms would alert the nurse to stop maraviroc therapy?

1. Re-current infections and respiratory distress
2. Itchy rash, yellow skin, dark urine, vomiting
3. Reduced hemoglobin levels and signs of bleeding
4. Increased white blood cell count and fever

Answers: Question 1(2), Question 2(2), Question 3 (3), Question 4(1,2,3), Question 5(2)

Study Strategy

This study guide differs from other resources because formal rationale is not provided for the answers. **You need to determine the appropriate rationale for the correct answers by accessing the information in the question that may have inhibited your ability to answer the question correctly.** It is helpful to ask the following questions:

- What is the question asking? What are key words in the question query?
- What information do I need to know to answer this question correctly?
- How did I select my answer?
- Why were the other answers incorrect?
- Was I missing a piece of content knowledge that inhibited how I answered the question? If so, what should I target in on and study?

Additional Strategies for Working with the Pharmacology Study Guide Modules

Content review is essential for being successful at answering NCLEX-RN® exam questions focusing on pharmacology. The following tips will help you to navigate the breath of this content and to organize your study notes. **Remember that you need to do the work of solid content review in order to be successful in understanding pharmacological concepts. Do not rely on practice questions to teach you what you need to know regarding medications for the NCLEX-RN®- practice questions are a tool for consolidating knowledge not a primary way to study.**

1. Complete the exercises in this study guide and make notes. This guide has been designed to direct you to important content for medication review.

When creating the study guide I used an educator's lens to pull out the most important information in order ensure client safety with drug administration. For example, when review differing drugs I focused on critical information and essential education for each drug. The review questions are designed to bring this information forward.

2. Find ways to colour code or organize medications according to the bodily system or pathology they are used for. This will help you with recalling information. This guide uses a systems approach to help you organize the vast amount of pharmacological review in a way that will help you understand key concepts and pathologies.
3. Create case studies or unique ways to remember classes of medications. It is always wise to study pharmacology in the context of pathology. Use case studies specifically for content that is new to you or more difficult. Case studies should be memorable, contain client information that is easy to remember, focus on adverse effects of medications and key aspects of client education.
4. It is helpful to find patterns in names in drugs- such as suffixes that are common. Highlight the endings of common terms and find strategies to remember the main side effects of these classes of medications.
5. Client teaching is essential in medication administration. Ensure that you review your client education chapter in your Fundamentals of Nursing textbook (e.g. Potter and Perry). You need to remember that the use of basic teaching and learning principles paired with your knowledge of medications can help you to better exam questions.
6. When you use practice questions find consistent strategies for reviewing questions that you get incorrect. For example, the summary drug tables presented in each module of this guide provide a structure for organizing information. Create a blank table with the drug classes named for each system. Write information or content that is tested in each drug class as you move through your practice resources. Highlight the medication names you have seen in the practice questions on your summary table. Are there any patterns in the types of questions asked or the content tested? **Do be careful with this strategy- it is not a replacement for reviewing content.**

Conclusion

Strong pharmacological review will not only increase your chances of success on the NCLEX-RN® it will also strengthen your future nursing practice. The complexity of client care paired with the increase in co-morbidity and chronic disease management poses many challenges to pharmacological therapy. Nurses must be aware of potential drug-to-drug interactions, polypharmacy, and adverse events related to medications in order to keep their clients safe. I wish you all the best for your NCLEX-RN® exam and for your future nursing practice.

Best wishes,

Dr. Marnie Kramer-Kile

REFERENCES

Copstead, L.E & Banaski, J. (2013). *Pathophysiology* (5th ed). St. Louis: Elsevier.

Richards, J.S. (2013). Overview of herbal supplements. *Elite Continuing Education*, 46-72.

Rosenjack Burchum, J. & Rosenthal, L.D. (2016). *Lehne's pharmacology for nursing care* (9th edition). St. Louis: Elsevier.

Module 8

Drugs Affecting the Endocrine System

TABLE OF CONTENTS

Introduction to the Transitioning to the NCLEX-RN® Pharmacology Guide: Drugs Affecting the Endocrine Medications

The breadth and detail of the knowledge required of pharmacological concepts often overwhelms new graduates when they are beginning their exam preparation. The purpose of this pharmacology study guide is to help you work through the vast amount of pharmacological knowledge required for the NCLEX-RN® in a systematic and purposeful way. This guide organizes content using the current NCLEX-RN® Test Plan and provides specific strategies to address pharmacological areas of review which may challenge new graduates. **This is the eighth of twelve modules.** This is a working guide, so while key information will be presented and organized for review, it is up to you to do the detailed work of content review by answering the questions and exercises in each section. You can expect to see drugs described by their generic names on the exam. Due to the differences in drug trade names between the United States of America, Canada and other nations you should study drugs according to their generic names and develop strategies for remembering them.

This module is part of a comprehensive pharmacology study guide focusing on specific areas which may challenge NCLEX-RN® candidates. This includes drug-to-drug interactions, specific adverse reactions due to drug therapy and the potential reactions associated with herbal therapy and conventional medications. The content will be focused on a systems approach and will direct you towards important information within each drug class.

Structure of the Module

This module begins with an overview of the drugs influencing the Endocrine System. Additional areas for review that are specialized or affect multiple systems will also be highlighted:

1. Review questions and selected exercises will be constructed for each drug class to help pull out key concepts such as adverse events/side effects, specific client teaching and drug to drug interactions.
2. A summary chart of the drug classes in each system or theme will be provided for you to use alongside practice questions. As you move through practice questions, check off the specific medications you come across and if you require further review in each area. It is also helpful to make your own drug cards for specific medications. Keep the drug cards simple. Identify the drug class, the mechanism of action, two relevant (i.e., life threatening) or unique adverse effects that require monitoring and provide an outline for client teaching or specific nursing interventions for the medication.

Advice for Studying Pharmacological Content for the NCLEX-RN®

Always start with areas you are NOT familiar with. For example, if you spent the majority of your time as a final practicum student/or nurse on a cardiology unit do not start in the Vascular and Cardiac Medications Module. It is common for students/graduates to move to areas of comfort when they are studying because it decreases their anxiety. However, your efforts should be targeted on what you don't know. Each Module in this guide has a summary table of drugs for each system. Highlight the drug classes that you are not familiar with and make it your priority to work through them. Do not spend time making drug cards for medications you already know. For example, most students are confident with furosemide administration and can critically think through concepts associated with the drug. Therefore, time does not need to be spent studying this medication. Only make drug cards for medications that are new to you. The review questions in this guide will direct you towards more detailed information of the medications that you are familiar with and focus on potential areas where exam questions may be asked.

This guide is set up using a **systems approach** for the following reasons: 1) most pharmacology textbooks use this approach to structure content so it will be easier to find the information you need to answer the review questions; 2) using a systems approach allows you to find commonalties in the side effects of drugs influencing a specific system, so you will see patterns arising as you work through this guide; and 3) a systems approach allows for the creation of overall drug summary tables, which will be included in each module of the guide and will provide you with a general sense of the medications you need to cover.

The following resources will aid you in answering questions posed in this guide. This includes:

1. **A pharmacology textbook.** This resource will contain more detailed information pertaining to drug classes and outline general nursing considerations for therapy. I have referenced a pharmacology textbook throughout the writing of this guide.
2. **A drug guide**. These are the guides commonly used for your clinical practice. These resources contain alphabetized drug information. Most importantly, they outline specific pharmacokinetic and pharmacodynamics properties of drugs. You will find information related to drug excretion, protein binding, and therapeutic index in these guides.
3. **An online drug repository** for more detailed information that may not be found in the two resources above. Sometimes it is difficult to find therapeutic index and protein binding for a drug. I have found the following website helpful for this: http://www.drugbank.ca/drugs

Module 8: Drugs Affecting the Endocrine System

Table 8.1: Drug Therapy for Diabetes Mellitus

Oral Drugs	**Oral Drugs**	**Non-Insulin Injectable Drugs**
Biguanide metformin **Second Generation Sulfonylureas** Glimepride Glipizide Glyburide **Meglitinides (Glinides)** Nateglinide Repaglinkide **Thiazolidinediones (Glitazones)** Pioglitazone Rosiglitazone	**Alpha-Glucosidase Inhibitors** Acarbose Miglitol **DPP-4 Inhibitors (Gliptins)** Alogliptin Linaliptin Saxagliptin Sitagliptin **Sodium-Glucose Co-Transporter 2 (SGLT-2) Inhibitors** Canagliflozin Dapagliflozin **Dopamine Agonist** Bromocriptine	**Incretin Mimetics** Exenatide Exenatide extended-release Liraglutide Albiglutide **Amylin Mimetics** Pramlintide
Insulin Short Duration: Rapid Acting Insulin lispro Insulin aspart Insulin glulisine	**Insulin Short Duration: Slower Acting** Regular insulin **Intermediate Duration** NPH insulin	**Long Duration** Insulin glargine Insulin detemire

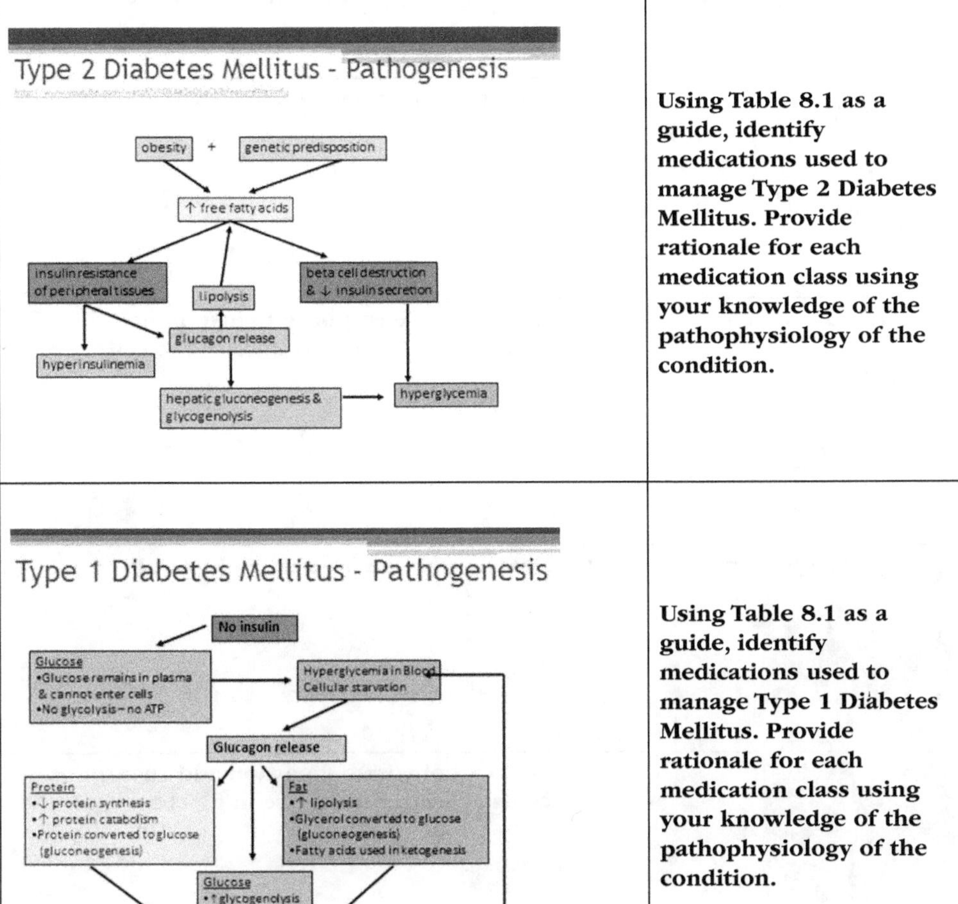

Using Table 8.1 as a guide, identify medications used to manage Type 2 Diabetes Mellitus. Provide rationale for each medication class using your knowledge of the pathophysiology of the condition.

Using Table 8.1 as a guide, identify medications used to manage Type 1 Diabetes Mellitus. Provide rationale for each medication class using your knowledge of the pathophysiology of the condition.

Table 8.2 Comparison Table for Oral Anti-Hyperglycemic Medications

Key to Figures:

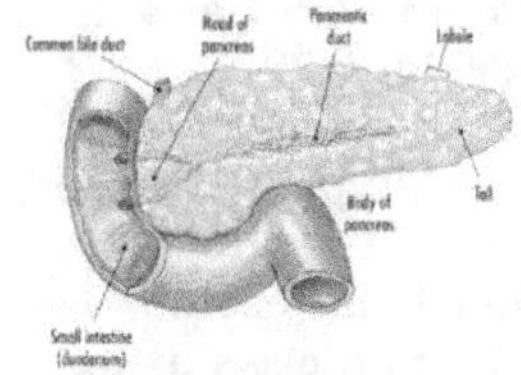	**Promotes Insulin Secretion by the Pancreas**
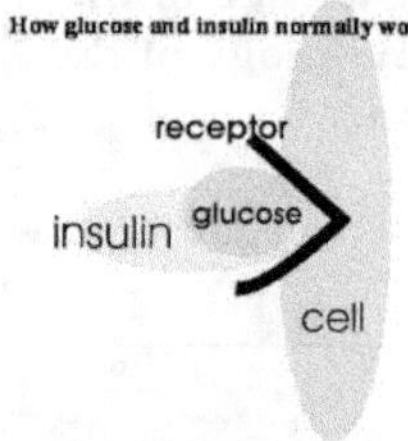	**Increases tissue response to insulin by descreasing insulin resistance in the cell**
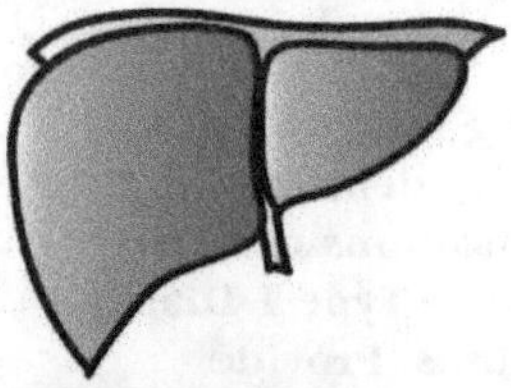	**Decreases glucose production by the liver**
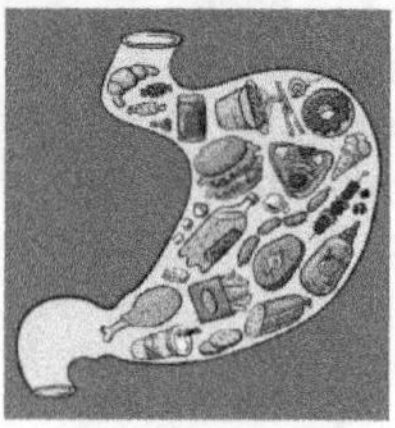	**Delays carbohydrate digestion and absorption—decreases postprandial rise in glucose**

Drug Class	Use in Type 1 or Type 2 DM	Mechanism of Drug Action	Causes Hypoglycemia	Major Side Effects	Nursing Considerations
Sulfonylureas (First and Second Generation Drugs)	Type 1: YES Type 2: YES	Act by stimulating release of insulin from pancreatic islet cells and by increasing the sensitivity of insulin receptors on target cells.	YES	Weight gain, hypersensitivity reactions, GI distress, hepatotoxicity. Second generation drugs have fewer drug-drug side effects.	Monitor when taking with alcohol as may cause flushing, palpitations and nausea
Biguanides (e.g., Metformin)	TYPE 1: NO TYPE 2: YES	Facilitates insulin's action on peripheral receptor sites (decreases hepatic production of glucose and reduces insulin resistance). Insulin must be present for drug to work, no effect on pancreatic beta cells.	NO	Lactic acidosis potential and serious S/E in pts with liver dysfunction.	Contraindicated in pts with renal impairment. Not given 2 days prior to contrast agent for DI. Interacts with anticoagulants, corticosteroids, diuretics and oral contraceptives.

Alpha-Glucosidase Inhibitors (e.g., Acarbose)	TYPE 1: NO TYPE 2: YES	Act by blocking enzymes in small intestine resp. for breaking down complex carbohydrates (delays digestion of glucose). Does NOT enhance insulin secretion	NO—when used alone. MAY INCREASE HYPOGLYCEMIA if used with insulin or sulfonylureas or with concurrent use of garlic or ginsing.	GI side effects: abdominal cramping, diarrhea and flatulence	Monitor liver function
Thiazolidinediones (e.g., rosiglitazone)	TYPE 1: NO TYPE 2: YES	Decreases insulin resistance/ inhibits hepatic gluconeogenesis. Enhances insulin action at the receptor site without increasing secretion of insulin from beta cells. Optimal lowering of therapy; may take 3-4 months	YES—but only in the presence of excessive insulin	Fluid retention, headache and weight gain	Can cause resumption of ovulation in perimenopausal anovulatory women, making pregnancy possible. May promote fluid retention, contraindicated for pts with heart failure or pulmonary edema. Monitor liver function

Meglitinides (e.g., repaglinide)	TYPE 1: NO TYPE 2: YES	Stimulates release of insulin from pancreatic beta cells similar to sulfonylureas Effectiveness depends on functioning beta cells	YES	Generally well tolerated with hypoglycemia major side effect	May be combined with metformin in pts whose hyperglycemia cannot be controlled by exercise, diet and either metformin or repaglinide alone. Should not take unless pt is eating a meal

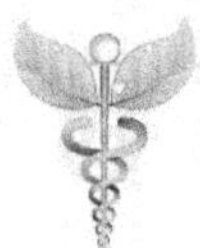

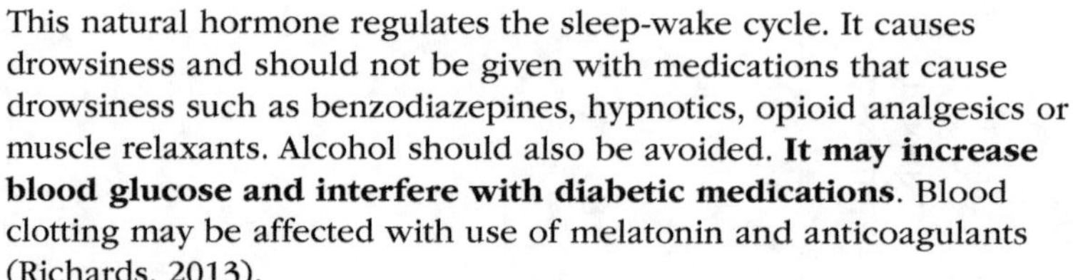

Integrative Therapy Caution

Herbal Medication: Melatonin

This natural hormone regulates the sleep-wake cycle. It causes drowsiness and should not be given with medications that cause drowsiness such as benzodiazepines, hypnotics, opioid analgesics or muscle relaxants. Alcohol should also be avoided. **It may increase blood glucose and interfere with diabetic medications**. Blood clotting may be affected with use of melatonin and anticoagulants (Richards, 2013).

REVIEW QUESTIONS

ORAL ANTIHYPERGLYCEMIC MEDICATIONS

1. Why does metformin have the risk of accumulating to toxic levels in clients with renal failure?
2. Why is metformin well suited for clients who often skip meals?
3. Is metformin safe to use in clients with gestational diabetes?
4. How does metformin work in women with polycystic ovary syndrome?
5. Which two vitamins does metformin decrease in the body?
6. Lactic acidosis is a rare side effect of metformin administration. Clients with liver disease, severe infection, history of lactic acidosis, alcohol abuse, shock or conditions that can result in hypoxemia are at the greatest risk when concurrently taking metformin. What are clinical signs of lactic acidosis? (Important note: Cimetidine and Iodinated Radiocontrast Media can increase incidences of lactic acidosis).
7. Identify drugs that are known to intensify hypoglycemia and should be avoided when administering sulfonylurea agents.
8. Repaglinide (a meglitinide drug) should never be administered with Gemfibrozil (a drug used to lower triglyceride levels). Why?
9. Why should pioglitazine (a thiazolidinedione) be used in caution with clients with Heart Failure? What are the links to this drug and bladder cancer? How does this drug affect plasma lipids?
10. Create a drug card for Sitagliptin (Dipeptidyl Peptidase-4 (DPP-4) Inhibitor). What type of hypersensitivity reaction has this drug been linked to?
11. Create a drug card for Canagliflozin (Sodium-Glucose Co-Transporter 2 (SGLT-2) Inhibitors). Explain the mechanism of action of this medication.

INSULIN

1. Complete the following table:

Generic Name of Insulin	Onset (min)	Peak (hr)	Duration (hr)
Insulin lispro			
Insulin aspart			
Insulin glulisine			
Regular insulin (e.g., Humulin R)			
NPH insulin (e.g., Humulin N)			
Insulin glargine			
Insulin detemir			

2. Which insulins can be administered via the IV route?
3. Which insulins can be mixed with other insulins?
4. Which insulins can be administered via a portable insulin pump?
5. Outline the complications related to insulin therapy. Ensure you address how to assess for and intervene for these complications.
6. Identify drugs that can LOWER blood glucose levels and INTENSIFY the effects of insulin.
7. Identify drugs that can RAISE blood glucose levels and COUNTERACT the desired effects of insulin.
8. Beta-blockers can delay awareness of and response to hypoglycemia in the body. How do they do this?

NON-INSULIN INJECTABLE AGENTS

1. Create a drug card for Exenatide (Glucagon-Like Peptide-1 Receptor Antagonist). Explain how it works in the body. It will cause hypoglycemia when combined with which oral antihyperglycemic drug?
2. Exenatide can cause pancreatic. What are signs and symptoms of this condition?
3. Exenatide delays gastric emptying and slows the oral absorption of other drugs. What will happen to peak plasma levels of these other drugs if absorption is inhibited? (oral drugs should be given 1 hour prior to Exenatide to stay these effects).
4. Pramlintide is an Amylin Mimetic, a new drug used to complement the effects of insulin in clients with Type 1 and 2 Diabetes Mellitus. Severe hypoglycemia is the biggest concern with this medication. Why?

Tips for answering exam questions related to medications for the treatment of diabetes: (Rosenjack Burchum et al., 2016, p. 698-702)

- Review the steps of administering insulin via the sc route and focus on client education
- Insulin when unopened is stored in the refrigerator until the expiry date on the vial
- Insulin vials in current use can be stored at room temperature for up to 1 month, but must be kept out of direct sunlight or direct heat. Discard partially filled vials after several weeks if left unused (p. 699).
- Insulin vials can be stored 1 month at room temperature and up to 3 months when refrigerated
- Prefilled insulin syringes must be stored vertically (needle pointing up) in the refrigerator for 1-2 weeks
- Review normal blood glucose levels and optimal levels for glycemic management
- Be prepared to recognize the signs and symptoms of hypoglycemia in an exam question
- Be familiar with medications (e.g., beta blockers) that may mask signs of hypoglycemia
- Alcohol use increases changes of lactic acidosis in clients taking metformin
- Be aware of the oral diabetic drugs that cause hypoglycemia
- Be familiar with signs of liver injury (n&v, abdominal pain, fatigue, anorexia, dark urine, jaundice)
- If any of the oral diabetic drugs have a life-threatening potential side effect, be aware of the signs and symptoms of it. (e.g., pioglitazone can potentially cause: heart failure, liver injury, bladder cancer, fractures, and cause ovulation in premenopausal women, increasing risk of pregnancy)

Recommended Study Resources

Canadian Diabetes Association Health Care Provider Tools: http://guidelines.diabetes.ca/healthcareprovidertools

***This website is amazing—use this section to supplement your studying and print off copies for your notes.**

Registered Nurses' Association of Ontario (2012). Assessment and management of foot ulcers for people with diabetes. Toronto: Author. Retrieved from http://rnao.ca/bpg/guidelines/assessment-and-management-foot-ulcers-people- diabetes

Registered Nurses' Association of Ontario (December, 2005). Diabetes and you. Toronto: Author. Retrieved from http://rnao.ca/bpg/fact-sheets/diabetes-you

Registered Nurses' Association of Ontario (2004). Reducing foot complications for people with diabetes. Toronto: Author. Retrieved from http://rnao.ca/bpg/guidelines/reducing-foot-complications-people-diabetes

EXERCISE 5:

The following chart contains questions to help you cover the required content for studying Diabetes Mellitus. Integrate your knowledge of the pharmacology into the review questions as appropriate.

Knowledge	Application	Critical Thinking
Define hypoinsulinemia. How do the counter-regulatory hormones regulate insulin? Explain the role of insulin and how it helps glucose to get into the cell. Risk factors for Type 1 diabetes. Risk factors associated with metabolic syndrome Diagnosis of type 1 diabetes (i.e., fasting blood glucose, HgA1C, random blood glucose, oral glucose tolerance tests) Identify the different insulin preparations.	Outline the pathophysiology related to Type 1 Diabetes How would a patient present if they had hypoglycemia? How would a patient present if they had hyperglycemia? Explain why prolonged hyperglycemia causes dehydration. Describe the diabetic ketoacidosis. Describe hyperglycemic non-ketotic coma. Explain why gestational diabetes is considered a prediabetes condition. Identify pertinent patient teaching related to metabolic syndrome. How do rapid, short, intermediate and long acting insulins differ in regards to their onset of action?	Describe the clinical presentation of a person with Type 1 and Type 2 Diabetes. Compare and contrast Somogyi effect and Dawn phenomenon. Describe potential microvascular complications related to diabetes (make a teaching plan for a patient in order to prevent and recognize these complications). Describe potential macrovascular complications related to diabetes (make a teaching plan for a patient in order to prevent and recognize these potential complications) Explain the relationship between diabetes and infection. What type of oral anti-hyperglycemic medications are prescribed to individuals with type 1 diabetes? Why?

What are the signs and symptoms of gestational diabetes? How is gestational diabetes diagnosed?	Insulin pumps use which kind of insulin? What is the only type of insulin that can be given through an IV route? What are the immediate nursing actions to take if a patient has been given too much insulin? Which medications are safe to administer to a pregnant woman with gestational diabetes?	A patient with a known history of diabetes is found unconscious. Should the nurse give insulin or glucagon (IM) if there was no way to obtain an immediate blood sugar? Provide rationale? Interpret a sliding scale. What type of insulin is typically used for a sliding scale?

Table 8.3 Drugs Influencing the Endocrine System

Thyroid Disorders **Hypothyroidism** Levothyroxine (T4) Liothyronine (T3) Liotrix **Hyperthyroidism** Antithyroid Drugs: Thionamides Radioactive Iodine Nonradioactive Iodine: Lugol's Solution Beta Blockers	**Hypothalmic and Pituitary Function** Mecasermin (Insulin-like growth factor-1) Prolactin Thyrotropin Adrenocorticotropin Hormone Gonadotropins Antidiuretic Hormone (Vasopressin) Antidiuretic Hormone (Vasopressin) Antagonists Oxytocin	**Drugs for Disorders of the Adrenal Cortex** **Glucocorticoids** Hydrocortisone Dexamethasone Prednisone Cortisone Fludrocortisone Cosyntropin
Menopausal Hormone Therapy **Estrogens** Conjugated estrogens Conjugated estrogens (synthetic) Estradiol Estradiol acetate Estropipate Ethinyl estradiol **Progestins** Drospirenone Hydroxyprogesterone caproate Levonorgestrel Medroxyprogesterone acetate Megestrol acetate Norethindrone Norethindrone acetate Norgestimate Norgestrel Progesterone	**Birth Control** Combination oral contraceptives Progestin-only oral contraceptives Transdermal contraceptive patch Vaginal Contraceptive ring Subdermal etonogestrel implants Depot medroxyprogesterone acetate Intrauterine devices Spermicides Barrier Devices **Drugs for Medical Abortion** Mifepristone with Misoprostol Methotrexate with Misoprostol Prostaglandins (misoprostol, carboprost, dinoprostone)	**Androgens** Fluoxymesterone Methyltestosterone Oxandrolone Testosterone Testosterone cypionate Testosterone enanthate **Drugs for Erectile Dysfunction** Sildenafil Vardenafil, Tadalafil, Avanafil Papverine plus phentolamine Alprostadil **Benign Prostatic Hyperplasia (BPH) Drugs** 5-Alpha-Reductase Inhibitors Alpha$_1$-Adrenergic Antagonists Alpha$_1$ Blocker/5-Alpha-reductase Inhibitor Combination Tadalafil

REVIEW QUESTIONS

THYROID DISORDERS

The key to understanding the pharmacologic treatment for thyroid disorders is to understand the role of T3 and T4 in stimulating the thyroid gland. Review concepts related to:

a. The three principal actions of the thyroid hormones
b. The effect of iodine deficiency on thyroid function
c. Thyroid function tests: Serum TSH, Serum T_4 Test, Serum T_3 Test (research the reference ranges and know which levels would alert the Health Care Provider re: hypo or hyperthyroidism)

HYPOTHYROIDISM

Hypothyroidism in adults requires replacement therapy with thyroid hormones, in most cases this is required as lifelong therapy (Rosenjack Burchum et al., 2016, p. 705). Standard treatment is with:

Levothyroxine (T4) or Combined therapy of levothyroxine (T4) plus liothyronine (T3). To date, combined T3/T4 offers no advantage over T4 because T4 is rapidly converted to T3 which is the active form of the hormone (p. 705).

1. Levothyroxine is highly protein bound and therefore has a long half-life. This is beneficial for achieving steady plasma levels long term, however, it takes time for these levels to rise to therapeutic levels. When teaching a client about new levothyroxine therapy, how long should they expect it to take for the medication to reach a steady state?
2. Acute overdose of levothyroxine can cause thyrotoxicosis. What are signs and symptoms of this condition?
3. Which drugs can decrease the absorption of levothyroxine? How long should doses of these drugs be spaced between levothyroxine administration?
4. Levothyroxine accelerates the degradation of vitamin K-dependent clotting factors. Which drug will levothyroxine administration influence as a result of this?
5. A client receiving levothyroxine becomes critically ill and requires the administration of catecholamines (e.g., dopamine, epinephrine, dobutamine). What is the client at risk for as a result of receiving these medications while still on levothyroxine?
6. Levothyroxine is most commonly given orally. It can be given IV in certain instances. Identify when IV administration may be indicated?
7. Research the following conditions associated with hypothyroidism: myxedema coma, cretinism, simple goiter

HYPERTHYROIDISM

Grave's disease is the most common cause of excessive thyroid hormone secretion. It is primarily treated with the surgical removal of thyroid tissue, destruction of thyroid tissue with radioactive iodine or treatment with antithyroid drugs (methimazole or proylthiouracil).

1. Methimazole is the first-line drug for hyperthyroidism. What is the mechanism of action of this drug? (*of interesting note: methimazole does not bind to plasma protein*)
2. What is the most dangerous side effect of methimazole administration? What are signs of this potentially fatal disorder?
3. Proylthiouracil has similar mechanisms of action to methimazole. However, it poses a risk of liver injury, especially in children. What would be signs that a client is suffering liver injury while taking this medication?
4. How is radioactive iodine administered? Why is its administration considered inappropriate in very young children?
5. What is Lugol's solution? How is it administered? What is iodism (identify the symptoms of this side effect)?
6. Why would a client with hyperthyroidism be prescribed beta blocker therapy? What is the most common beta blocker prescribed to clients with hyperthyroidism?

DRUGS RELATED TO HYPOTHALMIC AND PITUITARY FUNCTION

1. Growth hormones are administered to children (primarily) and occasionally in adults when the pituitary gland is under-producing these hormones. Two main drugs given are: somatropin and mecasermin. Make drug cards for each of these medications.
2. What is acromegaly? Drugs given for this condition include: octreotide and lanreotide and pegvisomant. Make drug cards for each medication. Octreotide has other indications for use, what are they?
3. When would Antidiuretic Hormone (Vasopressin) be administered? What are adverse effects associated with administration of this hormone?
4. Antidiuretic Hormone (Vasopressin) Antagonists block the effects of ADH in renal collecting ducts. Two drugs are available: conivaptan and tolvaptan. When would these drugs be administered?
5. What are indications for the administration of oxytocin. What must the nurse monitor while administering this hormone?

DRUGS FOR DISORDERS OF THE ADRENAL CORTEX

The adrenal cortex produces three classes of steroid hormones: 1) glucocorticoids, 2) mineralocorticoids and 3) androgens (Rosenjack Burchum et al., 2016, p. 725). Take time to review the role of each of these hormones to help you understand the pathophysiology of disorders of the adrenal cortex. Two major pathologies to study the administration of drugs in this class include:

A. **Cushing's syndrome**: adrenal hormone excess (treat the cause, ketoconazole may be used)
B. **Addison's disease**: adrenal insufficiency (hydrocortisone, fludrocortisone)

1. Why would ketoconazole, an antifungal drug, be indicated for the treatment of Cushing's syndrome? What is its mechanism of action on glucocorticoid synthesis? Which organ is potentially damaged with the administration of this drug?
2. Hydrocortisone therapy needs to be increased during times of stress. What is the "3 by 3 rule" when a client has a mild or febrile illness?
3. How should hydrocortisone be dosed daily?
4. Excessive doses of fludrocortisone can cause retention of sodium and water. Serum potassium levels may decrease as a result from excessive fluid volume. What other conditions can result from excessive fluid volume associated with this medication?

HORMONE REPLACEMENT THERAPY (HRT)

ESTROGENS

Women who have an intact uterus should receive estrogen plus progestin while women how have had a hysterectomy should use estrogen alone. In both cases estrogen is given daily and estrogen/progestin can be given daily or cyclically 10 days per month (Rosenjack Burchum et al., 2016, p. 749).

1. What are indications for estrogen replacement therapy? What baseline data should be collected before starting therapy?
2. What conditions would contraindicate estrogen administration?
3. Outline the client teaching required for administration of estrogen via the following routes:
   a. Transdermal Patch
   b. Transdermal Emulsion
   c. Transdermal Gel
   d. Transdermal Spray
   e. Intravaginal Cream
   f. Intravaginal Ring
   g. Intravaginal Tablet
4. Endometrial carcinoma is a risk with estrogen therapy. What are signs of this condition?
5. What should the nurse teach the client regarding screening for breast, lung and ovarian cancer while on HRT?
6. What specific teaching should the nurse provide to the client in regards to reducing cardiac risk while taking HRT?

PROGESTINS

Remember that progestins are given with estrogen in HRT. The role of progestins in menopause is to counteract endometrial hyperplasia that could be caused by unopposed estrogen during HRT. Progestins are contraindicated in the presence of undiagnosed vaginal bleeding.

1. What are the potential gynecologic effects of progestins?
2. Create drug cards for drospirenone and progesterone.

BIRTH CONTROL

1. There are two main categories of oral contraceptive medications. What are they and which hormones do each use?
2. What are adverse events associated with oral contraceptive use?
3. When should initial dosing of an oral contraceptive start? (it is important to note that depending on the oral contraceptive "days off" may differ)
4. What should the nurse teach the client regarding "missed doses" of oral contraceptives?
5. How soon can oral contraceptives be initiated after delivery in post-partum clients? How does breast-feeding influence this?
6. The most important concept in studying oral contraceptives is knowing which drugs "inactivate or reduce" the effects of oral contraceptives. Identify 3 medications that inactivate oral contraceptives.

Integrative Therapy Caution

Herbal Medication: Black Cohosh

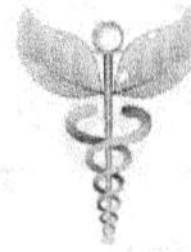

Black Cohosh is used for menopausal disorders, painful menstruation, uterine spasms and vaginitis. It may enhance liver toxicity with certain medications that also cause liver toxicity (e.g., atorvastatin, acetaminophen, alcohol). The common drug-to-drug interaction is drug toxicity because of liver impairment (Richards, 2013).

ANDOGRENS

1. What are indications for androgen therapy in males and females?
2. What should the nurse teach the client administering androgen therapy via the transdermal (gel & solution) and buccal routes?
3. What is virilisation and why would this occur in women taking androgen therapy?
4. What should the nurse teach the client regarding skin-to-skin transfer of androgen therapy to other individuals from the client?

DRUGS FOR ERECTILE DYSFUNCTION AND BENIGN PROSTATIC HYPERLASIA (BPH)

1. What are common adverse events associated with the use of Sildenafil?
2. What happens when Sildenafil is taken with: 1) Nitrates or 2) Alpha Blockers (e.g., doxazosin)?
3. What is the maximum daily dosage of Sildenafil?
4. Finasteride is used to treat BPH. What are precautions that pregnant women should take around this medication? Why are men not allowed to donate blood until 1 month after therapy has been stopped?
5. How does finasteride affect prostate-specific antigen (PSA) screening for prostate cancer?
6. $Alpha_1$-Adrenergic antagonists are also used to treat BPH. These drugs include terazosin, doxazosin, alfuzosin (non-selective) tamsulosin and silodosin (selective). What are common side effects of non-selective and selective $Alpha_1$-Adrenergic antagonists? Identify side effects that are specific to non-selective and selective $Alpha_1$-Adrenergic antagonists.

Integrative Therapy Caution

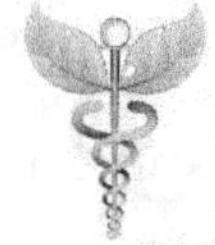

Herbal Medication: Saw Plametto

Used for BPH and noncancerous prostate gland enlargement. There is evidence that it may be effective for mild-to-moderate BPH. Do not give it with other medications used for BPH (e.g., finasteride). It slows blood clotting and may increase risk of bleeding if given with warfarin. It can also reduce the effectiveness of estrogens or oral contraceptives (Richards, 2013).

PRACTICE QUESTIONS

Question 1
A client is started on oral antihyperglycemic drug therapy for Type 2 diabetes. Which of the following drugs have the potential to cause hypoglycemia when given on their own? **(Select all that apply)**

1. Metformin 500mg po daily
2. Glyburide 2.5 mg po daily
3. Acarbose 25mg po tid
4. Rosiglitazone 4mg po daily
5. Repaglinide 0.5mg po tid

Question 2
A 52-year-old female client has been started on Rosigliazone for management of Type 2 Diabetes Mellitus. What is a critical piece of information for the nurse to teach a client taking this therapy?

1. Not to ingest the medication with alcohol because it causes an disulfiram-like reaction
2. There is the potential for the medication to have adverse reactions with oral contraceptives
3. The medication is to be discontinued during times of dehydration or illness
4. The medication can cause resumption of ovulation in perimenopausal anovulatory women

Question 3
A 62-year-old male client with Type 2 diabetes is admitted to the emergency room for a hypoglycemic episode. He takes an oral hypoglycemic medication and insulin regularly. His current blood glucose level is 2.5 mmol/L. The client's wife states that he does not recognize when his blood sugar drops to a critical level. Which of the following medications might be masking the client's hypoglycemic episodes?

1. Warfarin 2mg po daily
2. Ramipril 2.5 mg po bid
3. Metoprolol 25 mg po bid
4. Lispro insulin daily with meals

Question 4
A client is receiving levothyroxine therapy. The nurse is teaching the client regarding the signs and symptoms of thyrotoxicosis. Which of the following signs and symptoms are associated with this condition? **(Select all that apply)**

1. Tachycardia
2. Angina
3. Bradycardia
4. Hyperthermia
5. Sore throat

Question 5
A client is taking Methimazole. Which of the following symptoms would the nurse report to the Health Care Provider immediately?

1. Increased INR levels
2. Decreased WBC levels
3. Increased myoglobin levels
4. Decreased aPTT levels

Question 6
A client with Diabetes Insipidus is receiving Antidiuretic hormone (vasopressin). What is an expected effect of this medication for a client with this condition?

1. Decreased urine output
2. Increased urine output
3. Decreased edema
4. Increased blood pressure

Answers: Question 1(2,4,5), Question 2(4), Question 3 (3), Question 4(1,2,4), Question 5(2); Question 6(1)

Study Strategy

This study guide differs from other resources because formal rationale is not provided for the answers. **You need to determine the appropriate rationale for the correct answers by accessing the information in the question that may have inhibited your ability to answer the question correctly.** It is helpful to ask the following questions:

- What is the question asking? What are key words in the question query?
- What information do I need to know to answer this question correctly?
- How did I select my answer?
- Why were the other answers incorrect?
- Was I missing a piece of content knowledge that inhibited how I answered the question? If so, what should I target in on and study?

Additional Strategies for Working with the Pharmacology Study Guide Modules

Content review is essential for being successful at answering NCLEX-RN® exam questions focusing on pharmacology. The following tips will help you to navigate the breath of this content and to organize your study notes. **Remember that you need to do the work of solid content review in order to be successful in understanding pharmacological concepts. Do not rely on practice questions to teach you what you need to know regarding medications for the NCLEX-RN®- practice questions are a tool for consolidating knowledge not a primary way to study.**

1. Complete the exercises in this study guide and make notes. This guide has been designed to direct you to important content for medication review. When creating the study guide I used an educator's lens to pull out the most important information in order ensure client safety with drug administration. For example, when review differing drugs I focused on critical information and essential education for each drug. The review questions are designed to bring this information forward.
2. Find ways to colour code or organize medications according to the bodily system or pathology they are used for. This will help you with recalling information. This guide uses a systems approach to help you organize the vast amount of pharmacological review in a way that will help you understand key concepts and pathologies.
3. Create case studies or unique ways to remember classes of medications. It is always wise to study pharmacology in the context of pathology. Use case studies specifically for content that is new to you or more difficult. Case studies should be memorable, contain client information that is easy to remember, focus on adverse effects of medications and key aspects of client education.

4. It is helpful to find patterns in names in drugs- such as suffixes that are common. Highlight the endings of common terms and find strategies to remember the main side effects of these classes of medications.
5. Client teaching is essential in medication administration. Ensure that you review your client education chapter in your Fundamentals of Nursing text-book (e.g. Potter and Perry). You need to remember that the use of basic teaching and learning principles paired with your knowledge of medications can help you to better exam questions.
6. When you use practice questions find consistent strategies for reviewing questions that you get incorrect. For example, the summary drug tables presented in each module of this guide provide a structure for organizing information. Create a blank table with the drug classes named for each system. Write information or content that is tested in each drug class as you move through your practice resources. Highlight the medication names you have seen in the practice questions on your summary table. Are there any patterns in the types of questions asked or the content tested? **Do be careful with this strategy- it is not a replacement for reviewing content.**

Conclusion

Strong pharmacological review will not only increase your chances of success on the NCLEX-RN® it will also strengthen your future nursing practice. The complexity of client care paired with the increase in co-morbidity and chronic disease management poses many challenges to pharmacological therapy. Nurses must be aware of potential drug-to-drug interactions, polypharmacy, and adverse events related to medications in order to keep their clients safe. I wish you all the best for your NCLEX-RN® exam and for your future nursing practice.

Best wishes,

Dr. Marnie Kramer-Kile

REFERENCES

Copstead, L.E & Banaski, J. (2013). *Pathophysiology* (5th ed). St. Louis: Elsevier.

Richards, J.S. (2013). Overview of herbal supplements. *Elite Continuing Education*, 46-72.

Rosenjack Burchum, J. & Rosenthal, L.D. (2016). *Lehne's pharmacology for nursing care* (9th edition). St. Louis: Elsevier.

Module 9

Antineoplastic Medications

TABLE OF CONTENTS

Tables and Figures

Introduction to the Transitioning to the NCLEX-RN® Pharmacology Guide: Antineoplastic Medications

The breadth and detail of the knowledge required of pharmacological concepts often overwhelms new graduates when they are beginning their exam preparation. The purpose of this pharmacology study guide is to help you work through the vast amount of pharmacological knowledge required for the NCLEX-RN® in a systematic and purposeful way. This guide organizes content using the current NCLEX-RN® Test Plan and provides specific strategies to address pharmacological areas of review which may challenge new graduates. **This is the ninth of twelve modules.** This is a working guide, so while key information will be presented and organized for review, it is up to you to do the detailed work of content review by answering the questions and exercises in each section. You can expect to see drugs described by their generic names on the exam. Due to the differences in drug trade names between the United States of America, Canada and other nations you should study drugs according to their generic names and develop strategies for remembering them.

This module is part of a comprehensive pharmacology study guide focusing on specific areas which may challenge NCLEX-RN® candidates. This includes drug-to-drug interactions, specific adverse reactions due to drug therapy and the potential reactions associated with herbal therapy and conventional medications. The content will be focused on a systems approach and will direct you towards important information within each drug class.

Structure of the Module

This module begins with an overview of the drugs given for cancer treatment. Additional areas for review that are specialized or affect multiple systems will also be highlighted:

1. Review questions and selected exercises will be constructed for each drug class to help pull out key concepts such as adverse events/side effects, specific client teaching and drug to drug interactions.
2. A summary chart of the drug classes in each system or theme will be provided for you to use alongside practice questions. As you move through practice questions, check off the specific medications you come across and if you require further review in each area. It is also helpful to make your own drug cards for specific medications. Keep the drug cards simple. Identify the drug class, the mechanism of action, two relevant (i.e., life threatening) or unique adverse effects that require monitoring and provide an outline for client teaching or specific nursing interventions for the medication.

Advice for Studying Pharmacological Content for the NCLEX-RN®

Always start with areas you are NOT familiar with. For example, if you spent the majority of your time as a final practicum student/or nurse on a cardiology unit do not start in the Vascular and Cardiac Medications Module. It is common for students/graduates to move to areas of comfort when they are studying because it decreases their anxiety. However, your efforts should be targeted on what you don't know. Each Module in this guide has a summary table of drugs for each system. Highlight the drug classes that you are not familiar with and make it your priority to work through them. Do not spend time making drug cards for medications you already know. For example, most students are confident with furosemide administration and can critically think through concepts associated with the drug. Therefore, time does not need to be spent studying this medication. Only make drug cards for medications that are new to you. The review questions in this guide will direct you towards more detailed information of the medications that you are familiar with and focus on potential areas where exam questions may be asked.

This guide is set up using a **systems approach** for the following reasons: 1) most pharmacology textbooks use this approach to structure content so it will be easier to find the information you need to answer the review questions; 2) using a systems approach allows you to find commonalties in the side effects of drugs influencing a specific system, so you will see patterns arising as you work through this guide; and 3) a systems approach allows for the creation of overall drug summary tables, which will be included in each module of the guide and will provide you with a general sense of the medications you need to cover.

The following resources will aid you in answering questions posed in this guide. This includes:

1. **A pharmacology textbook.** This resource will contain more detailed information pertaining to drug classes and outline general nursing considerations for therapy. I have referenced a pharmacology textbook throughout the writing of this guide.
2. **A drug guide**. These are the guides commonly used for your clinical practice. These resources contain alphabetized drug information. Most importantly, they outline specific pharmacokinetic and pharmacodynamics properties of drugs. You will find information related to drug excretion, protein binding, and therapeutic index in these guides.
3. **An online drug repository** for more detailed information that may not be found in the two resources above. Sometimes it is difficult to find therapeutic index and protein binding for a drug. I have found the following website helpful for this: http://www.drugbank.ca/drugs.

Module 9: Antineoplastic Medications

Understanding anti-neoplastic therapy begins with an understanding of the normal cell cycle (http://www2.le.ac.uk/departments/genetics/vgec/diagrams/22-Cell-cycle.gif).

Anti-neoplastic therapy is either:

1. Cell cycle specific
2. Non-cell cycle specific

Cell cycle specific therapy is effective for rapidly growing tumors. The goal of this therapy is to induce cytotoxic effects in the M or S phase of the cell cycle. **Non-cell cycle specific therapy** is cytotoxic in any phase of the cell cycle. Therefore, this class of anti-neoplastic therapy is effective for slow growing tumours. Therapy for both classes of anti-neoplastic medications can be given intermittently (allowing healthy cells to repopulate between treatments) or in combination therapy (multiple drugs eliciting a greater kill rate of cancerous cells with less healthy cells killed, but with potentially more toxic effects resulting from drug therapy).

The Table 9.1 highlights the most common medications given for the treatment of cancer. Studying these medications can be overwhelming. Begin by differentiating the classes and select a prototype for each class. Use your pharmacology textbook to help you identify the most common drugs given. Look for commonalities in each class and pay close attention to the adverse effects of the medication. There is a summary table of common adverse effects related to antineoplastic therapy in this module- when you are studying drugs think about life threatening and unique side effects of the drug you are reviewing. It is also helpful to come up with ways to remember these concepts- try drawing pictures or making case studies to help you retain important information.

Table 9.1 Summary of Antineoplastic Medications

CELL CYCLE SPECIFIC **Effective against rapidly growing tumors**		
PLANT ALKALOIDS	**ANTIMETABOLITIES**	**TOPOISOMERASE-1 INHIBITORS**
VINCA ALKALOIDS Vinblastine sulfate (Velban) Vincristine sulfate (Oncovin) Vinorelbine tartrate (Navelbine) **TAXANES** Docetaxel (Taxotere) Paclitaxel (Taxol)	**Methotrexate (Folex)** Pemtrexed (Alimta) Azacitidine (Vidaza) Capecitabine (Xeloda) Cytarabine (Cytosar-U) Floxuridine (FUDR) Fluorouracil (5-FU) Gemcitabine (Gemzar) Cladribine (Leustatin) Fludarabine (Fludara) Mercaptopurine (Purinethol) Nelarbine (Arranon) Pentostatin (Nipent) Thioguanine (Lanvis)	Etiposide (VePesid) Irinotecan hydrochloride (Camptosar) Teniposide (Vumon) Topotecan hydrochloride (Hycamtin)
CELL CYCLE NONSPECIFIC **Effective against large, slowly growing tumors**		**HORMONES AND HORMONE ANTAGONISTS (non-cytotoxic)**
ALKYLATING AGENTS	**ANTITUMOUR ANTIBIOTICS**	**HORMONES**
NITROGEN MUSTARDS Chlorambucil (Leukeran) Cyclophosphamide (Cytoxan, Neosar) Estramustine (Emcyt) Ifosfamide (Ifex) Mechlorethamine (Mustargen) Melphalan (Alkeran) **NITROSOUREAS** Carmustine (BiCNU) Lomustine (CeeNU) Streptozocin (Zanosar)	Bleomycin (Blenoxane) Dactinomycin (Actinomycin-D) **Daunorubicin (Cerubidine)** **Doxorubicin (Adriamycin, Rubex)** Epirubicin (Ellence) Idarubicin (Idamycin) Mitomycin (Mutamycin) Mitoxantrone (Novantrone) Plicamycin (Mithramycin) Valrubicin (Valstar)	Dexamethasone (Decadron) Diethylstilbestrol (Stibestrol) Ethinyl estradiol (Estinyl) Fluoxymesterone (Halotesin) Medroxyprogesterone (Provera, Depo-Provera) Megestrol (Megace) Prednisone Testolactone (Teslac) Testosterone (Andro)

MISCELLANEOUS ALKYLATING AGENTS Busulfan (Myleran) Carboplatin (Paraplatin) Dacarbazine (DTIC-Dome) Oxaliplatin (Eloxatin) Procarbazine (Matulane) Temozolomide (Temodar) Thiotepa (Thioplex)		**HORMONE ANTAGONISTS** Abarelix (Plenaxis) Aminoglutethimide (Cytadren) Anastrozole (Arimidex) Bicalutamide (Casodex) Exemestane (Aromasin) Flutamide (Eulexin) Fulvestrant (Faslodex) Goserelin (Zoladex) Histrelin (Vantas) Letrozole (Femara) Letrozole (Femara) Leuprolide (Eligard) Nilutamide (Nilandron) **Tamoxifen citrate (Nolvadex)** Toremifene (Fareston)

Figure 9.2 Outline of Cancer Treatment

Each cancer will require a different type of treatment; cancer treatment is becoming highly individualized

Cancer Treatment

1. Antineoplastic drugs
2. Hormone therapy
3. Immunomodifiers
4. Radiation
5. Surgery

1. Antineoplastic Drugs

(also referred to as chemotherapy)

2 Major Types

↙ ↘

Cell cycle Specific	**Cell cycle Nonspecific**
(plant alkaloids, antimetabolities, topoisomerase-1 inhibitors)	(alkylating agents, antitumor antibiotics)

Intermittent vs. Combined therapy, dosage schedule, regional drug administration
Administering Chemotherapy (cytotoxic drug precautions, methods of administration)

Side Effects of Antineoplastic Therapy

Bone Marrow Depression, GI disturbances in epithelial lining, Nausea and Vomiting, Stomatitis, Alopecia, Reproductive Toxicities, hyperuricemia, local injury at site of administration, drug specific effects, cancer

2. Hormone administration

(glucocorticoids, androgens and antiandrogens, estrogens and antiestrogens, progestin)

Used to combat cancer cells by competing for receptor sites for hormones that are known to increase or cause cancer or are used to help with the side effects of other treatments.

Serious side effects can occur, such as secondary sex characteristics in the case of estrogen or androgen administration, or Cushing's syndrome in the case of glucocorticoids.

3. Immunomodifiers

(also referred to as biological response modifiers)

Help to alter the body's response to cancer; can give the body's cells cytotoxic properties to attack cancer cells.

4. Radiation

Affects DNA of rapidly growing cells, may be used to decrease tumor size, relieves symptoms in palliative cases.

May cause shedding of the skin, hair loss, stomatitis, dry mouth, change or loss of taste, decreased salivation, esophageal irritation, dysphagia, anorexia, nausea and vomiting, diarrhea; radiation may cause fatigue and tumor lysis.

5. Surgery

Depends on size and location of malignant tumor.
Post-operative complications may occur.

CURE = 100% Kill Rate

Combining Anti-Neoplastic Therapies: Important Considerations Regarding Toxicity

	Anticancer Effect	Toxicity Neutropenia	Toxicity Neuropathy
Drug A	++	++	0
Drug B	++	0	++
Drug A & B	++++	++	++

Anti-neoplastic therapies are often combined in order to elicit a maximum kill rate of cancer cells. However, when drugs are combined, their action may be increased but so will the toxic effects. In the above table, Drug A has neutropenic effects, when combined with Drug B that has neuropathic effects the client may have better clinical results but now is faced with two potentially severe toxic effects. **It is important to study the adverse effects and toxicities associated with cytotoxic medications**. *An understanding of these concepts will help you answer exam questions related to this complicated and often overwhelming class of medications.* The review questions in the first part of this module are designed to direct you to the most common and serious toxic effects of these drugs.

Dose-Limiting Toxicities

As medication doses are increased, so also is the risk for higher-level toxicities. Sometimes drugs are administered until the risks of toxic effects become too great. It becomes an integral part of nursing assessment to be aware of and continually assess for potential toxic effects. Organs that are commonly affected by anti-neoplastic therapy are the kidneys, liver and heart. Table 9.3 summarizes some of the common side effects of chemotherapy and identifies pertinent nursing interventions. Remember, it is almost impossible to memorize all of the drugs presented in this module. Work through the differing drug classes and focus on the adverse effects and toxicities related to the medications. You will see similarities arising as you work through the review questions.

Table 9.3 Nursing Interventions to Monitor and Manage the Side Effects of Chemotherapy (Antineoplastic Medications): Cytotoxic

Side Effect/Description of Side Effect	Key Assessments/ Monitoring Required	Nursing Interventions
Bone marrow depression		
• evidenced by decreased serum levels of neutrophils, thrombocytes, erythrocytes • pt at risk for infection, bleeding, anemia	• Monitoring blood cell counts frequently • Assess for signs and symptoms of infection (fever, may not show increase in WBC as pt. has low counts to begin with) report fever over 38.5 degrees C. Chills, diaphoresis, swelling, heat, pain and any pus or drainage noted on the body. • Ensure no contact with individuals with infection	• Protect patient from infection or injury • Adhering to neutropenic precautions (reverse isolation in private room, no fresh fruit/ vegetables/flowers) • Administration of G-CSF or erythropoietin depending on pts blood count. • Monitor for bleeding in urine, epitaxis, etc. • Use only electric razors • Aseptic technique for all invasive procedures • Daily v/s • Send off culture and sensitivity tests (blood, urine, sputum) if infection suspected. • Avoid rectal or vaginal procedures • Hand hygiene for patient • Assess IV sites for infection • Avoid IM injections • Avoid insertion of urinary catheters • Cleanse skin with chlorahexadine before venipuncture

GI Tract		
• Break down in epithelial lining, as these cells rapidly proliferate. • pt. at risk for stomatitis, diarrhea (due to inflammation of mucosal lining)	• Assess oral cavity daily • Pt to report burning or pain in mouth or pain with swallowing • If severe, assess gag reflex • May need topical anesthetic such as viscous lidocaine a custom mixed mouthwash (Akabutu's Mouthwash, developed by a doctor at the Cross Cancer Institute)	• Avoid commercial mouthwashes • Brush with soft toothbrush • Culture mouth if infection suspected • Provide liquid or pureed diet if severe • Administer analgesics as needed
Nausea and Vomiting		
• Stimulation of chemotherapy trigger zone in medulla. May persist up to 24 hrs after administration, but may also be delayed (48-72 hours). Caused by activation of CTZ of the medulla, stimulation of peripheral ANS pathways, stimulation of vestibular pathways, cognitive stimulation (Day et al., 2007, p.337).	• Assessing fluid status—BP, HR, O2 sats, intake and output, bloodwork (serum osmolarity), skin turgor, perfusion • Looking for signs and symptoms of dehydration • Monitoring electrolyte levels (Na, Cl, K, Ca) • Also ensure that it is not another cause such as constipation, GI irritation, electrolyte imbalance, radiation therapy, mediations or CNS metastasis	• Administering anti-emetics (ondansetron most commonly used serotonin blocker, metoclopromide most common dopamine receptor blocker) • May administer sedatives or corticosteroids before and after chemotherapy as needed • Relaxation, imagery techniques • Alternating patient's diet to include small frequent meals, bland foods, comfort foods • Managing stimulants that increase nausea (smells etc.) • Administering IV therapy if needed • Increasing fluid intake if pt. vomiting • Frequent oral hygiene

Alopecia		
• Hair loss that begins 7-10 days after onset of treatment; regeneration occurs 1-2 months after treatment stops	• Monitoring for skin integrity • Monitoring emotional and coping skills in individual experiencing hair loss	• Discuss potential hair loss and re-growth • Explore potential impact of hair loss on self-image • Prevent or minimize hair loss (Day et al., 2007, p. 345) • Prevent trauma to scalp • Explain that hair growth starts after therapy completed
Hyperuricemia		
• Increased cell death from chemotherapy results in formation of uric crystals. • Can cause injury to kidneys from rapid tumor lysis (presents as increased K and Phos in the system low levels of Ca)	• Monitor BUN, serum creatinine, electrolytes (patient may need to have hemodialysis) • Increased uric crystals can be secreted through skin (smells like urine), also makes skin very dry	• Ensure adequate hydration • Encourage alkalization of urine through diet • Can administer allopurinol to prevent buildup of uric acid • Assess for confusion
Local Tissue Injury		
• At IV site; can cause necrosis and sloughing of tissue. Vesicants are those agents that, if deposited into subcutaneous tissue, cause tissue necrosis and damage to underlying tendons, nerves and blood vessels. Only specially trained RNs and physicians can administer vesicants.	• Monitor IV site for patency, interstitial sites, swelling, redness and pain at site • Monitor for absence of blood return from IV catheter • Resistance to flow of IV fluid	• Stop IV infusion if there is swelling or pain at the site. • May sometimes apply ice to site • Inform physician immediately if you suspect that a chemotherapeutic agent is interstitial • Physician may inject neutralizing agent into sc tissue.

REVIEW QUESTIONS

ALKYLATING AGENTS

1. Cyclophosphamide is a nitrogen mustard, alkylating agent, that can be given PO or IV. It is a pro-drug. What does this mean? This drug can also cause hemorrhagic cystitis. What are symptoms of this condition and how is it treated?
2. Nitrosoureas are another class of alkylating agents, they are highly lipophilic and can penetrate the blood brain barrier. What type of cancers are these drugs used to treat?
3. A client is receiving carmustine (a nitrosourea agent). An adverse effect related to this medication is pulmonary fibrosis (in high cumulative doses). Why would a glucocorticoid medication be given in this instance along with carmustine?

PLATINUM COMPOUNDS

1. Cisplatin is highly emetogenic—what does this mean and how is this managed?
2. Cisplatin therapy can cause kidney damage. Extensive hydration and diuretic therapy are used to manage this adverse effect. Amifostine is a medication that is also given to reduce kidney damage. What is the mechanism of action of this medication?
3. Anaphylactic reactions are associated with Carboplatin. How soon after drug administration do these side effects occur and what is the treatment for anaphylaxis?

Tips for answering exam questions related to these medications (Rosenjack Burchum et al., 2016, p. 1225)

- These drugs may injure bone marrow, hair follicles, GI mucosa and germinal epithelium
- Blood dysrasias—neutropenia, thrombocytopenia and anemia are of greatest concern
- Nausea and vomiting occur with all these medications
- Several alkylating agents are vesicants and must be administered through a free flowing IV line

ANTIMETABOLITES

There are three classes of antimetabolites. Each class is identified and one prototype drug is listed with each class below:

1. Folic acid analogs (methotrexate)
2. Pyrimidine analogs (fluorouracil)
3. Purine analog (mercaptopurine)

1. What are toxicities associated with methotrexate therapy? What is leucovorin rescue and why is it used in a client undergoing methotrexate therapy?
2. Cytarabine is primarily given for Acute Myelogenous Leukemia. The liposomal formulation of this drug can cause arachnoiditis. What are signs of this condition?
3. Mercaptopurine is given as maintenance therapy for acute lymphocytic leukemia in children and adults. What are the toxicities associated with this drug?

ANTITUMOR ANTIBIOTICS

This class of medications are only used to treat cancer (not infections) because they injure cells through direct interaction with DNA (Rosenjack Burchum et al., 2016, p. 1230). IV is the most common route for these medications because they are poorly absorbed orally.

1. Doxorubicin (conventional) can cause acute and delayed injury to the heart. Outline what potential acute and delayed effects are and how the nurse would assess for them.
2. Doxorubicin (liposomal) was created to increase uptake in cancer cells and decrease uptake in normal cells. What are the major dose limiting toxicities associated with this medication?

MITOTIC INHIBITORS

These medications act during the "M" phase to prevent cell division.

1. Vinca alkaloids are made from the periwinkle plant. Two of the most important drugs include: **vincristine** and **vinblastine**. Outline the specific toxicities of each of these drugs.
2. What are the effects of **paclitaxel** on the heart?
3. Severe neutropenia develops in almost all clients receiving **docetaxel** and **cabazitaxel**. At what neutrophil level should this medication be held?

TOPOISOMERASE INHIBITORS

1. Identify dose-limiting toxicities of **topotecan** and **irinotecan**.
2. Hypotension can occur with rapid IV administration of Etoposide. How can hypotension be avoided? (*hint: it has to do with drug preparation*)

HORMONAL AGENTS, TARGETED DRUGS AND NONCYTOTOXIC ANTICANCER DRUGS

Complete the following table in order to review the Nursing Considerations/ Adverse Effects for common medications related to the treatment of Breast and Prostate cancer. The majority of these medications are non-cytotoxic (although pertinent cytotoxic medications have been included).

Drugs for Breast Cancer	Prototype Drug	Nursing Considerations/ Relevant Adverse Effects
Antiestrogens	Tamoxifen	
Aromatase Inhibitors	Anastrozole	
HER2 Antagonists	Trastuzumab	
Cytotoxic Drugs	Doxorubicin/ cyclophosphamide Paclitaxel	
Drugs to delay Skeletal Events	Denosumab Zoledronate	
Drugs for Prostate Cancer		
Gonadotropin-releasing hormone agonists	Leuprolide	
Gonadotropin-releasing hormone antagonists	Degarelix	
Androgen Receptor Blockers	Flutamide	
CYP17 Inhibitor	Abiraterone	
Cytotoxic Drugs	Docetaxel Cabazitaxel	
Drugs to stay skeletal events	Denosumab Zoledronate	
Patient-specific immunotherapy	Sipuleucel-T	

Tips for answering exam questions related to these medications (Rosenjack Burchum et al., 2016, p. 1264-1265)

- Tamoxifen is a prodrug that undergoes activation by hepatic CYP2D6
- SSRIs such as fluoxetine, paroxetine and sertraline (often taken to supress hot flashes) inhibit CYP2D6 and can prevent tamoxifen activation, increasing the risk of reoccurrence of breast cancer
- Taxmoxifen increases the risk of endometrial cancer and thromboembolism
- Anastrozole is more effective than tamoxifen and poses no risk of endometrial cancer
- When breast or prostate cancer metastasizes to bone it can cause hypercalcemia and fractures—this risk is reduced by the administration of denosumab and zoledronate

TARGETED ANTICANCER DRUGS

**Please note that this drug class has not been covered in this section.*

Common medications include:

Imatinib (Gleevec) and Rituximab (Rituxan). Targeted anticancer drugs bind with specific molecules to supress tumor growth. The majority of these drugs are antibodies that bind with specific antigens on tumor cells or they are small molecules that inhibit intracellular enzymes (Rosenjack Burchum et al., 2016, p. 1250).

PRACTICE QUESTIONS

Question 1
Which of the following laboratory results would be consistent with an increased risk for bleeding associated with antineoplastic therapy?

1. Low platelet count.
2. High eosinophil count.
3. Low white blood count.
4. High red blood cell count.

Question 2
Combination drug therapy is often more effective than single drug therapy in the treatment of cancer because:

1. The same phase of the cell cycle is attacked by both drugs
2. The drugs used have different side effects that counteract each other
3. Combining chemotherapy drugs could destroy a greater percentage of cancer cells
4. Combination treatment allows administration of each agent in excess of the toxic dosages

Question 3
A client with breast cancer is taking Tamoxifen is being assessed by the nurse. Which of the following medications should alert the nurse to a potential drug-to-drug interaction?

1. Sertraline
2. Lorazepam
3. Phenelzine sulfate
4. Atenolol

Question 4
Which of the following interventions best prevents kidney injury during the administration of methotrexate?

1. Frequent monitoring of creatinine and BUN
2. Administration of mucomyst currently with methotrexate
3. Alkalinzation of urine to promote drug excretion
4. Avoiding high dose therapy

Question 5
A client is receiving IV doxorubicin (conventional) for the treatment of non-Hodgkin's lymphoma. The nurse is administering the initial dose of the medication. Which of the following symptoms are associated to severe side effects of this medication?

1. Dysrhythmias and electrocardiogram changes
2. Nausea and vomiting
3. Numbness in hands and feet
4. Diarrhea

Question 6
A client is receiving an anti-neoplastic drug known to supress bone marrow production. Which of the following medications would be appropriate to give alongside this drug because it does NOT cause bone marrow supression?

1. Vincristine
2. Vinblastine
3. Doxorubicin
4. Mitomycin

Answers: Question 1(1), Question 2(3), Question 3 (1), Question 4(3), Question 5(1), Question 6(1)

Study Strategy

This study guide differs from other resources because formal rationale is not provided for the answers. You need to determine the appropriate rationale for the correct answers by accessing the information in the question that may have inhibited your ability to answer the question correctly. It is helpful to ask the following questions:

- What is the question asking? What are key words in the question query?
- What information do I need to know to answer this question correctly?
- How did I select my answer?
- Why were the other answers incorrect?
- Was I missing a piece of content knowledge that inhibited how I answered the question? If so, what should I target in on and study?

Additional Strategies for Working with the Pharmacology Study Guide Modules

Content review is essential for being successful at answering NCLEX-RN® exam questions focusing on pharmacology. The following tips will help you to navigate the breath of this content and to organize your study notes. **Remember that you need to do the work of solid content review in order to be successful in understanding pharmacological concepts. Do not rely on practice questions to teach you what you need to know regarding medications for the NCLEX-RN®- practice questions are a tool for consolidating knowledge not a primary way to study.**

1. Complete the exercises in this study guide and make notes. This guide has been designed to direct you to important content for medication review. When creating the study guide I used an educator's lens to pull out the most important information in order ensure client safety with drug administration. For example, when review differing drugs I focused on critical information and essential education for each drug. The review questions are designed to bring this information forward.
2. Find ways to colour code or organize medications according to the bodily system or pathology they are used for. This will help you with recalling information. This guide uses a systems approach to help you organize the vast amount of pharmacological review in a way that will help you understand key concepts and pathologies.
3. Create case studies or unique ways to remember classes of medications. It is always wise to study pharmacology in the context of pathology. Use case studies specifically for content that is new to you or more difficult. Case studies should be memorable, contain client information that is easy to remember, focus on adverse effects of medications and key aspects of client education.

4. It is helpful to find patterns in names in drugs- such as suffixes that are common. Highlight the endings of common terms and find strategies to remember the main side effects of these classes of medications.
5. Client teaching is essential in medication administration. Ensure that you review your client education chapter in your Fundamentals of Nursing textbook (e.g. Potter and Perry). You need to remember that the use of basic teaching and learning principles paired with your knowledge of medications can help you to better exam questions.
6. When you use practice questions find consistent strategies for reviewing questions that you get incorrect. For example, the summary drug tables presented in each module of this guide provide a structure for organizing information. Create a blank table with the drug classes named for each system. Write information or content that is tested in each drug class as you move through your practice resources. Highlight the medication names you have seen in the practice questions on your summary table. Are there any patterns in the types of questions asked or the content tested? **Do be careful with this strategy- it is not a replacement for reviewing content.**

Conclusion

Strong pharmacological review will not only increase your chances of success on the NCLEX-RN® it will also strengthen your future nursing practice. The complexity of client care paired with the increase in co-morbidity and chronic disease management poses many challenges to pharmacological therapy. Nurses must be aware of potential drug-to-drug interactions, polypharmacy, and adverse events related to medications in order to keep their clients safe. I wish you all the best for your NCLEX-RN® exam and for your future nursing practice.

Best wishes,

Dr. Marnie Kramer-Kile

REFERENCES

Copstead, L.E & Banaski, J. (2013). *Pathophysiology* (5th ed). St. Louis: Elsevier.

Richards, J.S. (2013). Overview of herbal supplements. *Elite Continuing Education*, 46-72.

Rosenjack Burchum, J. & Rosenthal, L.D. (2016). *Lehne's pharmacology for nursing care* (9th edition). St. Louis: Elsevier.

Module 10

Medications Given in Mental Health Contexts

TABLE OF CONTENTS

Introduction to the Transitioning to the NCLEX-RN® Pharmacology Guide: Medications Given in Mental Health Contexts

The breadth and detail of the knowledge required of pharmacological concepts often overwhelms new graduates when they are beginning their exam preparation. The purpose of this pharmacology study guide is to help you work through the vast amount of pharmacological knowledge required for the NCLEX-RN® in a systematic and purposeful way. This guide organizes content using the current NCLEX-RN® Test Plan and provides specific strategies to address pharmacological areas of review which may challenge new graduates. **This is the tenth of twelve modules.** This is a working guide, so while key information will be presented and organized for review, it is up to you to do the detailed work of content review by answering the questions and exercises in each section. You can expect to see drugs described by their generic names on the exam. Due to the differences in drug trade names between the United States of America, Canada and other nations you should study drugs according to their generic names and develop strategies for remembering them.

This module is part of a comprehensive pharmacology study guide focusing on specific areas which may challenge NCLEX-RN® candidates. This includes drug-to-drug interactions, specific adverse reactions due to drug therapy and the potential reactions associated with herbal therapy and conventional medications. The content will be focused on a systems approach and will direct you towards important information within each drug class.

Structure of the Module

This module begins with an overview of the drugs given in the context of Mental Health. Additional areas for review that are specialized or affect multiple systems will also be highlighted:

1. Review questions and selected exercises will be constructed for each drug class to help pull out key concepts such as adverse events/side effects, specific client teaching and drug to drug interactions.
2. A summary chart of the drug classes in each system or theme will be provided for you to use alongside practice questions. As you move through practice questions, check off the specific medications you come across and if you require further review in each area. It is also helpful to make your own drug cards for specific medications. Keep the drug cards simple. Identify the drug class, the mechanism of action, two relevant (i.e., life threatening) or unique adverse effects that require monitoring and provide an outline for client teaching or specific nursing interventions for the medication.

Advice for Studying Pharmacological Content for the NCLEX-RN®

Always start with areas you are NOT familiar with. For example, if you spent the majority of your time in clinical practice administering SSRI antidepressants to clients do not start with this medication class in your preparation. It is common for students/graduates to move to areas of comfort when they are studying because it decreases their anxiety. However, your efforts should be targeted on what you don't know. Each Module in this guide has a summary table of drugs for each system. Highlight the drug classes that you are not familiar with and make it your priority to work through them. Do not spend time making drug cards for medications you already know. Only make drug cards for medications that are new to you. The review questions in this guide will direct you towards more detailed information of the medications that you are familiar with and focus on potential areas where exam questions may be asked.

This guide is set up using a **systems approach** for the following reasons: 1) most pharmacology textbooks use this approach to structure content so it will be easier to find the information you need to answer the review questions; 2) using a systems approach allows you to find commonalties in the side effects of drugs influencing a specific system, so you will see patterns arising as you work through this guide; and 3) a systems approach allows for the creation of overall drug summary tables, which will be included in each module of the guide and will provide you with a general sense of the medications you need to cover. The following resources will aid you in answering questions posed in this guide. This includes:

1. **A pharmacology textbook.** This resource will contain more detailed information pertaining to drug classes and outline general nursing considerations for therapy. I have referenced a pharmacology textbook throughout the writing of this guide.
2. **A drug guide**. These are the guides commonly used for your clinical practice. These resources contain alphabetized drug information. Most importantly, they outline specific pharmacokinetic and pharmacodynamics properties of drugs. You will find information related to drug excretion, protein binding, and therapeutic index in these guides.
3. **An online drug repository** for more detailed information that may not be found in the two resources above. Sometimes it is difficult to find therapeutic index and protein binding for a drug. I have found the following website helpful for this: http://www.drugbank.ca/drugs

Module 10: Medications Given in Mental Health Contexts

This module focuses on medications given specifically for anxiety disorders, depressive disorders, mood disorders and schizophrenia. Many of these medications are used for multiple disorders. Once you have a sense of the major drug classes and their mechanisms of action you may move towards studying individual drugs in more detail. **The following approach is recommended for this content**:

1. Review the pathophysiological mechanisms related to **anxiety**, **depression** and **mood disorders** in your nursing textbooks.
2. Review the role of the following **neurotransmitters** in the brain: **serotonin**, **dopamine** and **norepinephrine**. What happens when these neurotransmitters are blocked or inhibited at the synaptic site?
3. Start by familiarizing yourself with the drug classes. Ensure that you are aware of which drugs are first line agents for treatment.
4. Highlight on the summary drug charts any side effects that stand out in each drug class.
5. Answer the review questions provided for each drug class in this section. They will highlight any specific pieces of important information or client education.
6. Make specific drug cards for each medication listed on the drug summary table. Include the following on your card: 1) drug class; 2) mechanism of action; 3) <u>two</u> side effects that stand out; and 4) specific teaching interventions.
7. As you work your way through different practice question resources, keep track of the medication questions in this topic area. Write down key content areas being tested and see if you can recognize any patterns in the content being tested.

Study Strategy

There are life threatening complications related to some antipsychotics, antidepressants and mood stabilizers. **Start by gaining an**

understanding of these potential complications, signs and symptoms and their treatment. Examples include: Serotonin syndrome, neuroleptic malignant syndrome, hypertensive crisis, EPS symptoms, agranulocytosis, dehydration in clients taking Lithium.

Table 10.1: Drugs for the Treatment of Anxiety and Depression (Halter et al., 2014, 220-221)

Antidepressants	Antidepressants	Antidepressants
Selective Serotonin Reuptake Inhibitors Escitalopram oxalate (Cipralex) Fluoxetine hydrochloride (Prozac) Fluvoxamine maleate (Luvox) Paroxetine hydrochloride (Paxil) Sertraline hydrochloride (Zoloft) **Notable Side Effects:** agitation, insomnia, sexual dysfunction, hyponatremia, headache, nausea & vomiting Can cause Serotonin Syndrome (increase risk when these drugs are administered with another serotonin-enhancing agent)	Selective Serotonin-Norepinephrine Reuptake Inhibitors Duloxtine hydrochloride (Cymbalta) Venlafaxine hydrochloride (Effexor XR) **Notable Side Effects:** Hypertension, dry mouth, sexual dysfunction, sweating, agitation, nausea & vomiting, headache Monoamine Oxidase Inhibitors Phenelzine sulfate (Nardil) Tranylcypromine sulfate (Parnate) **Notable Side Effects:** Hypertensive crisis, serotonin syndrome with concurrent use of other antidepressants, insomnia, nausea, agitation, confusion	Tricyclics Amitriptyline hydrochloride (Elavil) Clomipramine hydrochloride (Anafranil) Desipramine hydrochloride (Norpramin) Doxepin hydrochloride (Adapin, Sinequan) Imipramine hydrochloride (Tofranil) Nortiptyline hydrochloride (Tofranil) Nortripyline hydrochloride (Tofranil) Nortiptyline hydrochloride (Aventyl, Norventyl) **Notable Side Effects:** Urinary retention, blurred vision, orthostatic hypotension, cardiac toxicity, sedation, dry mouth, constipation, weight gain
Antianxiety Agents Benzodiazepines Alprazolam (Xanax) Chlordiazepoxide hydrochloride (Librax) Clonazepam (Rivotril) Diazepam (Valium) Lorazepam (Ativan) Oxazepam (Serax)	**Antianxiety Agents** Nonbenzodiazepines Buspirone hydrochloride (Bustab) Anticonvulsants Carbamazepine (Tegretol) Gabapentin (Neurontin) Valproic acid (Depakote)	**Other Classes** Antihistamines Hydroxyzine hydrochloride (Atarax) Hydroxyzine pamoate (Vistaril) B-Blockers Atenolol (Tenormin) Propanolol (Inderal)

Table 10.2: Drugs for the Treatment of Clients with Major Depression (Halter et al., 2014, p. 245-246)

Most Common First Line Agents due to Decreased Side Effects and Low Lethality Risk when Overdosed:

Selective Serotonin Reuptake Inhibitors (SSRIs)	Serotonin-Norepinephrine Reuptake Inhibitors (SNRIs)	Tricyclics
Escitalopram oxalate (Cipralex) Fluoxetine hydrochloride (Prozac) Fluvoxamine maleate (Luvox) Paroxetine hydrochloride (Paxil) Sertraline hydrochloride (Zoloft) Citalopram (Celexa) **Notable Side Effects:** agitation, insomnia, sexual dysfunction, hyponatremia, headache, nausea & vomiting • Can cause Serotonin Syndrome (increase risk when these drugs are administered with another serotonin-enhancing agent)	Duloxtine hydrochloride (Cymbalta) Venlafaxine hydrochloride (Effexor XR) **Notable Side Effects:** Hypertension, dry mouth, sexual dysfunction, sweating, agitation, nausea & vomiting, headache. Monoamine Oxidase Inhibitors Phenelzine sulfate (Nardil) Tranylcypromine sulfate (Parnate) Moclobemide (Aurorix, Manerix) **Notable Side Effects:** Hypertensive crisis, serotonin syndrome with concurrent use of other antidepressants, insomnia, nausea, agitation, confusion	Amitriptyline hydrochloride (Elavil) Clomipramine hydrochloride (Anafranil) Nortiptyline hydrochloride (Aventyl, Norventyl) **Notable Side Effects:** Urinary retention, blurred vision, orthostatic hypotension, cardiac toxicity, sedation, dry mouth, constipation, weight gain Can cause dysrhythmias, tachycardia, myocardial infarction and heart block-not used in cardiac clients. Use of MAOI and tricyclics is contraindicated.
Norepinephrine Reuptake Inhibitors (NRIs) **Notable Side Effects:** urinary hesitancy, tachycardia, decreased libido, insomnia, sweating, dizziness, dry mouth	Norpinephrine Dopamine Reuptake Inhibitors (NDRIs) Bupropion (Wellbutrin)-also used for smoking cessation **Notable Side Effects:** Seizures (0.4%), agitation, insomnia, headache, nausea/vomiting	Serotonin Norepinephrine Disinhibitors (SNDIs) Mirtazpine (Remeron) **Notable Side Effects:** weight gain, sedation, dizziness, headache (sexual dysfunction is rare)

Review of Key Concepts for Medications Used to Treat Anxiety and Depression

There are 3 hypothesis of the mechanism of action of antidepressant drug therapy (Gutierrez, Raynor & Swart, 2014, p. 62-63).

1. **Monoamine Hypothesis of Depression:** There is a deficiency of one or more of the following three neurotransmitters: dopamine, serotonin, norepinephrine. The theory is that increasing these neurotransmitters alleviates depression.
2. **Monoamine Receptor Hypothesis of Depression:** Low levels of neurotransmitters causes postsynaptic receptors to be more sensitive. When neurotransmitter availability is increased by antidepressant therapy, these same receptors can become less sensitive and take longer to take up neurotransmitters at the synaptic site. This is the reason why antidepressant therapy takes so long to work effectively.
3. **Increase production of neurotrophic factors with prolonged use:** These factors are responsible for regulating the survival of neurons and the sprouting of new axons for synaptic connections. Therefore, antidepressant therapy is thought to increase the availability of synaptic connections for neurotransmitters, hence causing increased uptake and alleviating depressive symptoms.

All Antidepressant Drugs work to increase the availability of one or more of the neurotransmitters: serotonin, norepinephrine or dopamine (Halter et al., 2014, p. 244). All classes work equally well but a combination may need to be tried for individual clients.

Integrative Therapy Caution

Herbal Medication: Valerian

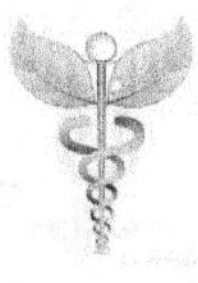

Used to treat insomnia and anxiety. It has over 500 possible drug interactions. It should be used with caution when combining it with muscle relaxants, sleep or anxiety medications, pain medications or antidepressants (Richards, 2013).

SELECTIVE SEROTONIN REUPTAKE INHIBITORS

How Do Antidepressants Work? YouTube Video: https://www.youtube.com/watch?v=G4r3qCkLUDQ

Block the reuptake and, thereby, the destruction of serotonin. Recommended as first line agents for antidepressant therapy.

1. Why are SSRI's less lethal than other antidepressant drug classes when taken as an overdose?
2. What are other indications for SSRI's besides the treatment of depression?
3. What are the effects on sexual performance associated with SSRI therapy?

Serotonin Syndrome

Which drug classes put a client at risk for developing serotonin syndrome?

What are the signs of this condition?

How long should a client who discontinues SSRI therapy wait until starting a second serotonin-enhancing agent? (e.g., MAOI)?

TRICYCLIC ANTIDEPRESSANTS

These drugs act by **blocking the re-uptake of *norepinephrine*** for secondary amines and of both norepinephrine and ***serotonin*** for the tertiary amines—more simply put, this blocking action prevents norepinephrine from being broken down (degraded) by MAO and increases the levels of norepinephrine at the synapse (Halter et al., 2010, p. 63). Some tricyclic medications also block Histamine-1 receptors, thereby causing sedation and drowsiness.

Tricyclic antidepressants have many different types of interactions with other drugs. Start by familiarizing yourself with common drugs in this class—you can recognize them by their generic name in that they all end with "hydrochloride."

Drugs to use with caution with Tricyclic Antidepressants

Complete the following table:

Drug Class	Example of Drug	Potential Interaction Occurring
Monoamine oxidase inhibitors		
Phenothiazines		
Barbiturates		
Oral contraceptives (or other estrogen preparations)		
Anticoagulants		
Anithypertensives (clonidine, guanethidine, reserpine)		
Benzodiazepines		
Alcohol		
Nicotine		

1. How is a tricyclic drug overdose treated?
2. What are common adverse reactions due to these drugs and which ones do you think are the most responsible for non-adherence in clients?
3. How long does it take for TCA drugs to start working?
4. Tricyclic drugs can be stimulating or sedating. Identify which specific drugs in the TCA class are stimulating and sedating.
5. Why should the dose be started low and then increased?
6. Think about the side effects listed with TCA's in summary drug charts above define which of the following symptoms are:
   a. Anticholinergic actions
   b. Due to alpha-adrenergic blockage
7. Why is the total daily dose of TCA drugs given at nighttime?
8. Can TCA drugs be given with MAO Inhibitors?
9. Why can't clients with a cardiac history be given these medications?
10. Should the initial symptoms of drowsiness, dizziness and hypotension subside after the client has been on medications for a few weeks?
11. Can clients drink alcohol while on these medications?
12. Should these medications be stopped suddenly? Why or why not?

MONOAMINE OXIDASE INHIBITORS

Monoamine is an enzyme responsible for breaking down monoamine neurotransmitters in the brain such as norepinephrine, serotonin, dopamine and tyramine. MAOI drugs make sure these amines do not get inactivated and there is an increase in all of these above neurotransmitters. This works for depression because of the treatment of norepinephrine, serotonin and dopamine. However, the problem becomes the increased amounts of tyramine this can lead to high blood pressure, hypertensive crisis and CVA (p. 248).

1. Which medical conditions contraindicate the use of MAOI therapy?
2. Is hypotension a normal adverse reaction to MAOIs? How should hypotension be assessed with this type of therapy?
3. Create a teaching plan regarding diet planning for a client on MAOI therapy (Hint: it is helpful to list foods that contain tyramine and create practice multiple response questions focused on these concepts).
4. What are the cardinal signs that a client is experiencing hypertensive crisis related to MAOI therapy?
5. If a client is experiencing a toxic effect of MAOI therapy such as hypertensive crisis what should the nurse advise them to do?
6. Identify two common drugs given to lower a client's blood pressure when they are experiencing hypertensive crisis related to MAOI therapy.

Integrative Therapy Caution

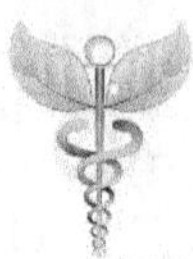

Herbal Medication: Yohimbe

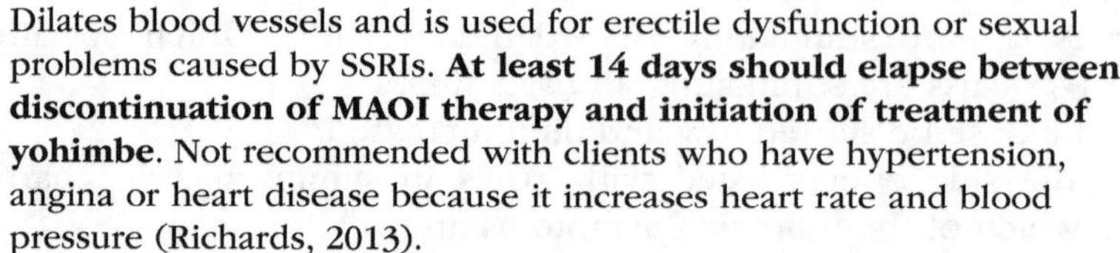

Dilates blood vessels and is used for erectile dysfunction or sexual problems caused by SSRIs. **At least 14 days should elapse between discontinuation of MAOI therapy and initiation of treatment of yohimbe**. Not recommended with clients who have hypertension, angina or heart disease because it increases heart rate and blood pressure (Richards, 2013).

SEROTONIN-NOREPINEPHRINE REUPTAKE INHIBITORS (SNRIS)

These medications increase both serotonin and norepinephrine in the synaptic site:

1. Duloxetine hydrochloride treats major depressive order as well as which other disorders?
2. Some SNRIs are also used to treat neuropathic pain. What is the mechanism of action of this effect?
3. Venlafaxine hydrochloride (Effexor XR) works as a SSRI at lower doses and a SNRI at higher doses. Why?

SEROTONIN AND NOREPINEPHRINE DISINHIBITORS

There is only one drug in this class: Mirtazapine (Remeron)—this drug increases norepinephrine, dopamine and serotonin transmission by blocking central pre-synaptic alpha 2-adrenergi c inhibitory receptors. It has both antianxiety and antidepressant effects.

1. Mirtazapine is a potent histamine (H_1) receptor antagonist which causes drowsiness and increased appetite. Why does this happen?
2. Is this class of drug authorized for use in children?
3. What are potential symptoms if this medication is discontinued abruptly?

ANXIETY SPECIFIC MEDICATIONS

These medications are used to treat somatic and psychological symptoms of anxiety, the goal of these medications is to help the client reduce their anxiety enough to participate in treatment of any underlying problems (p. 219). Clients with substance abuse problems can be given antihistamines as a non-addictive alternative to benzodiazepines to lower anxiety levels (p. 222).

BENZODIAZEPINES

1. Benzodiazepines have a quick onset of action. However, they should only be used for a short period of time due to risk of dependence. What are common adverse effects of these medications?
2. Why should women who are seeking to get pregnant NOT be given benzodiazepines?
3. Identify potential drug interactions that can occur with benzodiazepines.
4. Cessation of benzodiazepines after 3-4 months of daily use will cause withdrawal symptoms. Identify symptoms of withdrawal.

OTHER CLASSES OF MEDICATIONS TO TREAT ANXIETY

1. Propranolol and Atenolol are commonly prescribed to treat social anxiety disorder. What is the mechanism of action of these medications? Are they selective or non-selective beta blockers? How will this determine possible adverse effects?
2. Anticonvulsants such as carbamazepine, gabapentin and valporic acid are also used to treat anxiety disorders? What is the mechanism of action of these medications in the context of anxiety management?

Integrative Therapy Caution

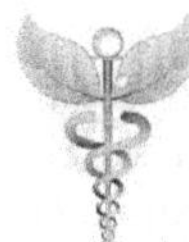

Herbal Medication: Kava Kava

Kava kava is marketed as an herbal sedative with antianxiety effects. **It is known to dramatically inhibit a liver enzyme necessary for the metabolism of medications and can result in liver failure, especially when taken with CNS depressants.** While it may be beneficial for short term management of anxiety, it is important to assess if clients are taking this medication. **The use of buprenorphine with kava can lead to respiratory distress or coma** (Richards, 2013).

Integrative Therapy Caution

Herbal Medication: St. John's

St. John's Wort should NOT be combined with: SSRI'S, TCAs, MAOIs, nefazodone, triptans for migraines, dextromethorphan, warfarin, birth control pills and certain HIV medications (Richards, 2013).

Table 10.3 Drugs for the Treatment of Clients with Mood Disorders

LITHIUM	ANTICONVULSANT DRUGS
Inhibits 80% of manic episodes within 10 to 21 days (p.270). It requires time to reach therapeutic levels in the blood. Antipsychotic or benzodiazapines may be given to prevent exhaustion, circulatory collapse and death until lithium is at a therapeutic level. Therapeutic levels of lithium are close to toxic levels- so careful monitoring and teaching is required. If lithium levels exceed 1.5-2 mmol/L the drug should be discontinued and if appropriate resumed at a lower level after 24 hrs. Excreted by the kidney, adequate fluid and salt intake are required	*Treatment of manic episodes refractory to lithium therapy for clients who require rapid descalation. Carbamazepine (Tegretol)- acute mania Valporic Acid (Depakene)- acute mania Lamotrigine (Lamictal)- maintenance medication
Drug Treatment of Clients with Mood Disorders (Halter, Watkins & Ray, 2014)	
OTHER TREATMENT RELATED TO BIPOLAR DISORDER Divalproex sodium (Epival)- maintenance medication Carbamazepine (Tegretol)- acute mania Lamotrigine (Lamictal)- maintenance medication	**ATYPICAL ANTIPSYCHOLTICS** Used for both manic and depressive phases of bipolar disorder- have sedative properties during early treatment but also act as mood-stabilizers Olanzapine (Zyprexa)- mania, maintenance Risperidone (Risperdal)- mania (first line treatment for severe mania) Aripiprazole (Abilify)- mania, maintenance Quetiapine (Seroquel)- depression, mania, maintenance Ziprasidone (Zeldox)- acute mania, mixed features

REVIEW QUESTIONS

LITHIUM

1. At what time of day should blood be drawn for lithium levels? How long should it be since the last dose?
2. Fill in the following table outlining the signs of lithium toxicity:

Serum Blood Level	Signs and Symptoms	Nursing Interventions
Expected Adverse Effects <0.4-1.0 mEq/L (therapeutic level)		
Early Signs of Toxicity < 1.5 mEq/L		
Advanced Signs of Toxicity 1.5-2.0 mEq/L		
Severe Toxicity 2.0-2.5 mEq/L < 2.5 mEq/L		

3. Low sodium intake results in lithium retention in the body, which can in turn produce toxicity. What is the recommended intake of salt and fluid intake for a client on lithium therapy?
4. What should a client do if they have excessive diarrhea, vomiting or sweating- or at risk of dehydration?
5. Can lithium therapy be abruptly discontinued?

OTHER MEDICATIONS FOR THE TREATMENT OF BIPOLAR DISORDER

1. Divalproex sodium is useful for lithium non-responders. However, it can also reach toxic levels. What are the therapeutic serum levels for this drug?
2. Cabamazepine (Tegretol) levels are to be monitored because it can increase levels of liver enzymes that can speed its own metabolism- so it is important to monitor for an increase in liver enzymes. Platelet levels and sodium levels should also be monitored, why?
3. Lamotrigine (Lamictal) is a first line treatment for bipolar depression but it has one severe (and rare) dermatological reaction—what is this reaction and how should the nurse assess for this?
4. Two serve drug to drug interactions are:
   a. Lamotrigine-valporic acid
   b. Carbamazepine-hormonal contraceptives
      - Explore what happens when these drugs are combined and explain the symptoms they produce.

Table 10.4: Drugs for the Treatment of Clients with Schizophrenia

<table>
<tr><td>1st Line Treatment Atypical Antipsychotics
Referred to as 2nd Generation Drugs

These drugs have fewer EPS symptoms and treat both positive and negative symptoms of schizophrenia (Halter, 2014)
They act by blocking dopamine
There are risks with these drugs which include:
Increased risk of metabolic syndrome (weight gain, dyslipidemia, altered glucose metabolism) which increases the risk of diabetes, hypertension and atherosclerotic heart disease.

Clozapine (Clozaril)- can cause agranulocytosis, high risk for metabolic syndrome</td><td>The following drugs are free of hematological adverse effects and have a low adverse effects profile.
Risperidone (Risperdal)
Quetiapine (Seroquel)
Olanzapine (Zyprexa)- high risk for metabolic syndrome
Ziprasidone (Zeldox)- does not cause metabolic syndrome
Aripiprazole (Abilify)- does not cause metabolic syndrome
Lurasidone (Latuda)</td></tr>
<tr><td colspan="2">Drug Treatment of Clients with Schizophrenia (Halter et al., 2014)</td></tr>
<tr><td>Conventional Antipsychotics

1st Generation Antipsychotic Drugs
Strong antagonists of dopamine 2 receptors, block the attachment of dopamine and decrease dopaminergic transmission, as a result they also block acetylcholine and alpha 1 adrenergic receptors for norepinephrine
• Dopamine blockage leads to EPS symptoms and increased release of prolactin
• Blockage of muscarinic receptors (a type of acetylcholine receptors) results in: blurred vision, dry mouth, constipation, urinary hesitancy and memory impairment
• Blockage of Alpha 1 Receptors can lead to: hypotension
• There are also Alpha 1 Receptors on the vas deferens blockage of these receptors from these drugs can cause a failure to ejaculate.
• Blockage of H1 receptors can lead to sedation and weight gain</td><td>Chlorpromazine
Loxapine (Loxapac0
Perphenazine
Thiothixene (Navane)
Fluphenaine (Modecate)
Haloperidol (Haldol)
Pimozde (Orap)
Flupentixol (Fluanxol, Fluanxol Depot)
Zuclopenthixol (Clopixol, Clopixol Depot, Clopixol Acuphase)</td></tr>
</table>

REVIEW QUESTIONS AND EXERCISES

1. Complete the following table focused on adverse effects of conventional antipsychotic therapy

Adverse Effect	Nursing Interventions to Treat Adverse Effect
Dry mouth	
Urinary retention and hesitancy	
Blurred vision	
Photosensitivity	
Impotence in men	
Anticholinergic-induced delirium	
Pseudoparkinsonism	
Acute dystonic reactions	
Opisthotonos	
Oculogyric crisis	
Laryngeal dystonia	
Akathisia	
Tardive dyskinesia	
Hypotension & postural hypotension	
Tachycardia	
Agranulocytosis	
Neuroleptic Malignant Syndrome	
Cholestatic jaundice	

2. Review the following medications for the treatment of antiparkinsonian and anticholinergic agents for the treatment of extrapyramidal side effects:
   a. Trihexyphenidyl (Apo-Trihex, Artane)
   b. Bentropine mesylate (Cogentin)
   c. Diphenhydramine hydrochloride (Benadryl)
3. Clozapine (Clozaril) has an increased risk of agranulocytosis in 0.8% to 1% of clients taking the medication (Halter et al., 2014, p.303). What type of monitoring do clients who take this drug require?

Integrative Therapy Caution

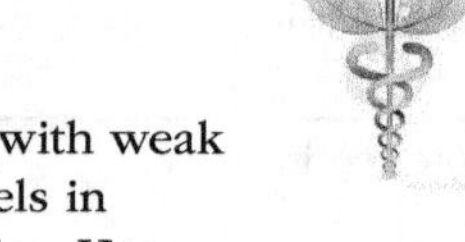

Herbal Medication: Goldenseal

Used for skin infections, cold and flu, treatment of diarrhea (with weak evidence in all categories). May raise antipsychotic blood levels in clients taking pimozide or thioridazine leading to dysrhythmias. Has over 60 differing drug interactions (Richards, 2013)..

PRACTICE QUESTIONS

Question 1
A client taking sertraline (Zoloft) has developed serotonin syndrome. Which of the following interventions should the nurse expect the health care provider to order to treat the client? **(Select all that apply)**:

1. Stop the medication
2. Administer propranolol
3. Treat hyperthermia with cooling blankets
4. Administer dantrolene
5. Encourage fluid intake

Question 2
Which of the following clients would the administration of Amitriptyline hydrochloride be contraindicated in?

1. Client with a history of major depression
2. Client diagnosed with severe anxiety
3. Client with a cardiac history and recent myocardial infarction
4. Client undergoing antineoplastic therapy

Question 3
A client is showing symptoms of hypertensive crisis related to MAO Inhibitor therapy. Which of the following medications should the nurse expect to administer to the client at this time?

1. Labetalol 10mg IV
2. Ramipril 5mg po
3. Candesartan 4mg po
4. Furosemide 40mg IV

Question 4
A client reveals that he is taking St. John's Wort to supplement his antidepressant therapy. What should the nurse teach the client regarding this herbal supplement?

1. St. John's Wort cannot be combined with most antidepressants
2. St. John's Wort has toxic effects to the Central Nervous System
3. St. John's Wort is safe to use as a supplement to conventional medical therapy
4. St. John's Wort may also interfere with blood clotting

Question 5
A client is admitted to the Emergency Department with a lithium level of 2.5 mEq/L. What symptoms should the nurse expect to assess for with a lithium level at this range?

1. High output of diluted urine, serious ECG changes, seizures, severe hypotension
2. Nausea, vomiting, diarrhea, thirst
3. Course hand tremor, confusion, incoordination
4. Convulsions, oliguria and possibility death

Question 6
Which of the following lab values would alert the nurse to one of the serious adverse events associated with the administration of Clozapine?

1. K+ 3.4 mmol/L
2. WBC 2 x 10^9/L
3. Neutrophil 7.5 x 10^9/L
4. International normalized ratio (INR) 1.2

Answers: Question 1(1,2,3,4), Question 2(3), Question 3 (1), Question 4(1), Question 5(1), Question 6(2)

Study Strategy

This study guide differs from other resources because formal rationale is not provided for the answers. **You need to determine the appropriate rationale for the correct answers by accessing the information in the question that may have inhibited your ability to answer the question correctly.** It is helpful to ask the following questions:

- What is the question asking? What are key words in the question query?
- What information do I need to know to answer this question correctly?
- How did I select my answer?
- Why were the other answers incorrect?
- Was I missing a piece of content knowledge that inhibited how I answered the question? If so, what should I target in on and study?

Additional Strategies for Working with the Pharmacology Study Guide Modules

Content review is essential for being successful at answering NCLEX-RN® exam questions focusing on pharmacology. The following tips will help you to navigate the breath of this content and to organize your study notes. **Remember that you need to do the work of solid content review in order to be successful in understanding pharmacological concepts. Do not rely on practice questions to teach you what you need to know regarding medications for the NCLEX-RN®- practice questions are a tool for consolidating knowledge not a primary way to study.**

1. Complete the exercises in this study guide and make notes. This guide has been designed to direct you to important content for medication review. When creating the study guide I used an educator's lens to pull out the most important information in order ensure client safety with drug administration. For example, when review differing drugs I focused on critical information and essential education for each drug. The review questions are designed to bring this information forward.
2. Find ways to colour code or organize medications according to the bodily system or pathology they are used for. This will help you with recalling information. This guide uses a systems approach to help you organize the vast amount of pharmacological review in a way that will help you understand key concepts and pathologies.
3. Create case studies or unique ways to remember classes of medications. It is always wise to study pharmacology in the context of pathology. Use case studies specifically for content that is new to you or more difficult. Case studies should be memorable, contain client information that is easy to remember, focus on adverse effects of medications and key aspects of client education.

4. It is helpful to find patterns in names in drugs- such as suffixes that are common. Highlight the endings of common terms and find strategies to remember the main side effects of these classes of medications.
5. Client teaching is essential in medication administration. Ensure that you review your client education chapter in your Fundamentals of Nursing textbook (e.g. Potter and Perry). You need to remember that the use of basic teaching and learning principles paired with your knowledge of medications can help you to better exam questions.
6. When you use practice questions find consistent strategies for reviewing questions that you get incorrect. For example, the summary drug tables presented in each module of this guide provide a structure for organizing information. Create a blank table with the drug classes named for each system. Write information or content that is tested in each drug class as you move through your practice resources. Highlight the medication names you have seen in the practice questions on your summary table. Are there any patterns in the types of questions asked or the content tested? **Do be careful with this strategy- it is not a replacement for reviewing content.**

Conclusion

Strong pharmacological review will not only increase your chances of success on the NCLEX-RN® it will also strengthen your future nursing practice. The complexity of client care paired with the increase in co-morbidity and chronic disease management poses many challenges to pharmacological therapy. Nurses must be aware of potential drug-to-drug interactions, polypharmacy, and adverse events related to medications in order to keep their clients safe. I wish you all the best for your NCLEX-RN® exam and for your future nursing practice.

Best wishes,

Dr. Marnie Kramer-Kile

REFERENCES

Copstead, L.E & Banaski, J. (2013). *Pathophysiology* (5th ed). St. Louis: Elsevier.

Gutierrez, M.A., Raynor, J. & Swart, B. (2014). Psychotropic drugs. In M.J. Halter, C.L. Pollard, S.L. Ray, M. Haase (2014). *Varcarolis's Canadian psychiatric mental health nursing: A clinical approach* (1st Canadian ed.). Toronto: Elsevier.

Halter, M.J., Pollard, C.L., Ray, S.L. & Haase, M. (2014). *Varcarolis's Canadian psychiatric mental health nursing: A clinical approach* (1st Canadian ed.). Toronto: Elsevier.

Richards, J.S. (2013). Overview of herbal supplements. *Elite Continuing Education*, 46-72.

Rosenjack Burchum, J. & Rosenthal, L.D. (2016). *Lehne's pharmacology for nursing care* (9th edition). St. Louis: Elsevier.

Module 11

Drugs and the Intra/Ante/Post-Partum Client

TABLE OF CONTENTS

Tables and Figures

Introduction to the Transitioning to the NCLEX-RN® Pharmacology Guide: Drugs and the Intra/Ante/Post-Partum Client

The breadth and detail of the knowledge required of pharmacological concepts often overwhelms new graduates when they are beginning their exam preparation. The purpose of this pharmacology study guide is to help you work through the vast amount of pharmacological knowledge required for the NCLEX-RN® in a systematic and purposeful way. This guide organizes content using the current NCLEX-RN® Test Plan and provides specific strategies to address pharmacological areas of review which may challenge new graduates. **This is the eleventh of twelve modules.** This is a working guide, so while key information will be presented and organized for review, it is up to you to do the detailed work of content review by answering the questions and exercises in each section. You can expect to see drugs described by their generic names on the exam. Due to the differences in drug trade names between the United States of America, Canada and other nations you should study drugs according to their generic names and develop strategies for remembering them.

This module is part of a comprehensive pharmacology study guide focusing on specific areas which may challenge NCLEX-RN® candidates. This includes drug-to-drug interactions, specific adverse reactions due to drug therapy and the potential reactions associated with herbal therapy and conventional medications. The content will be focused on a systems approach and will direct you towards important information within each drug class.

Structure of the Module

This module begins with an overview of the drugs given for intra/ante/post-partum clients. Additional areas for review that are specialized or affect multiple systems will also be highlighted:

1. Review questions and selected exercises will be constructed for each drug class to help pull out key concepts such as adverse events/side effects, specific client teaching and drug to drug interactions.
2. A summary chart of the drug classes in each system or theme will be provided for you to use alongside practice questions. As you move through practice questions, check off the specific medications you come across and if you require further review in each area. It is also helpful to make your own drug cards for specific medications. Keep the drug cards simple. Identify the drug class, the mechanism of action, two relevant (i.e., life threatening) or unique adverse effects that require monitoring and provide an outline for client teaching or specific nursing interventions for the medication.

Advice for Studying Pharmacological Content for the NCLEX-RN®

Always start with areas you are NOT familiar with. This module contains a summary table of drugs given during labor. Start by highlighting the drug classes that you are not familiar with and make it your priority to work through them. Do not spend time making drug cards for medications you already know. For example, most students are confident with morphine administration and can critically think through concepts associated with the drug. Therefore, time does not need to be spent studying this medication. Only make drug cards for medications that are new to you. The review questions in this guide will direct you towards more detailed information of the medications that you are familiar with and focus on potential areas where exam questions may be asked.

This module focuses specifically on pharmacological therapy related to pregnancy, the pregnant woman experiencing hypertension/gestational diabetes and the woman experiencing labor/complications related to childbirth. These areas commonly require further study and review because nursing graduates often have limited exposure to antepartum units in regards to medication administration. This module is designed to guide you towards pertinent content related to medication therapy in each of these areas. It is recommended that you review healthy pregnancy, stages of labor and post-partum assessment in order to have a strong foundation of what is "normal" so that you can advance to recognizing and treating complications with pharmacological therapy.

The following resources will aid you in answering questions posed in this guide. This includes:

1. **A pharmacology textbook.** This resource will contain more detailed information pertaining to drug classes and outline general nursing considerations for therapy. I have referenced a pharmacology textbook throughout the writing of this guide.
2. **A drug guide**. These are the guides commonly used for your clinical practice. These resources contain alphabetized drug information. Most importantly, they outline specific pharmacokinetic and pharmacodynamics properties of drugs. You will find information related to drug excretion, protein binding, and therapeutic index in these guides.
3. **An online drug repository** for more detailed information that may not be found in the two resources above. Sometimes it is difficult to find therapeutic index and protein binding for a drug. I have found the following website helpful for this: http://www.drugbank.ca/drugs

Module 11: Drugs and the Intra/Ante/Post-Partum Client

This module focuses on medications given during pregnancy, labor and the post-partum period. The focus is primarily on treating medical conditions during pregnancy that have the potential to harm the mother or the fetus and the management of acute complications occurring during and after labor.

GESTATIONAL HYPERTENSION

Gestational hypertension is the most common complication of pregnancy. It is defined as hypertension that was present before pregnancy or develops before the 20th week of gestation (p.513). Severe hypertension is generally treated with medication (SBP above 160 mmHg or DBP mmHg over 110) whereas mild hypertension (SBP 140-19 mmHg and DBP 90-109 mmHg). Methyldopa and labetalol are drugs of choice for treating chronic hypertension of pregnancy (p.515).

Drugs that must be discontinued if taken prior to the pregnancy include: Ace Inhibitors, Angiotensin Receptor Blockers, and Direct Renin Inhibitors because these drug classes can cause fetal harm.

It is important to remember not to aggressively drop blood pressure because it can cause limited uteroplacental blood flow.

REVIEW QUESTIONS

1. Identify at least **two drugs** in the following drug classes that are **contraindicated** for the treatment of gestational hypertension: Ace Inhibitors, Angiotensin Receptor Blockers, and Direct Renin Inhibitors.
2. What are adverse effects associated with labetalol administration?
3. How is labetalol dosed for the treatment of severe gestational hypertension?
4. Methyldopa can cause hemolytic anemia and hepatotoxicity as potential adverse effects. What is a Coombs' test and why would it be ordered for a client receiving this medication? What lab tests would confirm that hepatotoxicity is occurring?
5. What are clinical signs that confirm the presence of preclampsia? What are medications of choice for treating this condition? (please note that delivery of the baby is indicated for severely preclamptic mothers).
6. What is the medication of choice for treating eclampsia? How is it dosed and what are potential side effects?

GESTATIONAL DIABETES

Rosenjack Burchum et al. (2016, p.670) outline three factors that contribute to gestational diabetes in pregnant women:

1. Placenta produces hormones that antagonize insulin's actions
2. Cortisol production increases threefold during pregnancy
3. Hyperglycemia in the mother stimulates excessive secretion of insulin in the fetus

REVIEW QUESTIONS

1. Which oral antihyperglycemic medications are safe to administer during pregnancy?
2. How often should blood glucose testing be completed in mothers with gestational diabetes?
3. How is gestational diabetes diagnosed?
4. Do mothers have to continue with medication or insulin therapy post-delivery of the baby?

If a mother **has type 2 diabetes prior to pregnancy** the practice is to discontinue any oral antihyperglyemic therapy and put the mother on insulin (p.670). The only exception is for mothers who are taking metformin- this medication is typically continued during pregnancy for women who already have type 2 diabetes. After delivery the mother is taken off insulin and put back on oral antihyperglycemic therapy (p.670).

Table 11.1 Medications Administered During Labor (Hogan, 2012, p. 123, 837, 838).

Pain Management during Labor	
Medication	Nursing Assessment/Implications (identify routes of administration and any critical side effects or assessments required with the drug therapy)
Intravenous Opioids (morphine, fentanyl)	
Intrathecal Opioids (morphine, fentanyl)	
Lumbar Epidural Block	
Paracervical Block	
Pudendal Block	
Induction of Labor	
Medication	Nursing Assessment/Implications (identify routes of administration and any critical side effects or assessments required with the drug therapy)
Oxytocin (Pitocin)	
Misoprostol (Cytotec)	
Prostaglandin gel (PGE2)	

Drugs Used to Supress Pre-Term Labor (tocolytics—to stop contractions)	
Medication	Nursing Assessment/Implications (identify routes of administration and any critical side effects or assessments required with the drug therapy)
Ritodrine (Yutopar)	
Terbutaline (Brethine)	
Magnesium sulfate (evidence is declining for its use)	
Nifedipine	
Indomethacin	
Nitroglycerin	

Drugs used to Prevent Preterm Labor	
Medication	Nursing Assessment/Implications (identify routes of administration and any critical side effects or assessments required with the drug therapy)
Hydroxyprogesterone Caproate	

In the Event of Postpartum Hemorrhage	
Medication	Nursing Assessment/Implications (identify routes of administration and any critical side effects or assessments required with the drug therapy)
Oxytocin (Pitocin)	
Methylergonovine maleate (Methergine)	
Ergonovine maleate (ergotrate)	

Carboprost Tromethamine (Hemabate)	
Misoprostol	
Post-partum Infections	**Reproductive tract infections (i.e. metritis, parametrial cellulitis, peritonitis, septic pelvic thrombophlebitis, bacteremia and septic shock), wound infections, breast infections, urinary tract infections**
The type of anti-infective used will depend on the infective organism	The following link identifies common antibiotics that can be given during breastfeeding. However, if a mother's infection requires an antibiotic that may harm the baby through breastfeeding she may need to stop. http://www.drugs.com/drug-safety-breastfeeding.html

REVIEW QUESTIONS

DRUGS USED TO SUPPRESS PRETERM LABOR

According to Rosenjack Burchum et al. (2016) the goal of treatment of these medications is to extend fetal time in the womb without causing significant fetal or neonatal harm. Tocolytics work by promoting uterine relaxation, however, these drugs only suppress labor briefly (typically 48 hrs) so the birth typically takes place before term. When these drugs are combined with glucocorticoid medications they accelerate fetal lung development (p. 777). Magnesium sulfate has the ability to supress contractions by inhibiting the release of acetylcholine at the neuromuscular junction but it will not delay delivery. High dose magnesium sulfate administration has been shown to increase infant mortality because it can cause profound muscle weakness and respiratory arrest (p. 780).

1. Terbutaline is a $Beta_2$ -Adrenergic Agonist used primarily for asthma. What is the mechanism of action of this drug in the uterus? What are the potential harms to the mother who is taking this drug to suppress labor?
2. What are possible fetal harms or adverse effects from terbutaline?
3. Why would nifedipine, a CCB, be sued to suppress labor?
4. Indomethacin is considered a second-line tocolytic agent reserved for women who go into labor extremely early (p. 780). What are potential adverse fetal effects of this medication?
5. Nitroglycerin can also be used to suppress preterm labor. By what route is the nitroglycerin given? What are possible side effects in the mother and fetus of this medication?

Tips for answering exam questions related to these medications (Rosenjack Burchum et al., 2016):

- These medications promote uterine relaxation and thereby delay labor but only for a short period of time
- None of the drugs used to supress preterm labor have actually been approved for this specific use by the FDA
- Terbutaline, nifedipine, indomethacin and nitroglycerin are all used to suppress pre-term labor, there is no preferred first line agent
- Focus on the potential adverse effects of each of these medications on the mother and the fetus (particularly those medications that can cause hemodynamic instability)

DRUGS USED TO PREVENT PRETERM LABOR

Hydroxyprogesterone Caproate is the only drug approved by the FDA to prevent preterm labor. It is used in women with singleton pregnancies and a history of at least one preterm birth (Rosenjack Burchum et al., 2016, p. 780). The underlying mechanism of this drug is not known and it only works for some women.

1. By what route is this medication given?
2. What are noted adverse side effects?
3. Which client populations is this drug contraindicated in?

Tips for answering exam questions related to these medications (Rosenjack Burchum et al., 2016):

- Only women with singleton pregnancies and a history of one preterm labor birth qualify for this medication (p.780)
- Glucose intolerance, clinical depression and fluid retention can occur with this medication
- The medication is viscous and oily and must be injected slowly via IM route (healthcare providers, not clients, should administer this medication)

DRUGS FOR CERVICAL RIPENING AND THE INDUCTION OF LABOR

1. What are indications for early induction of labor?
2. What are contraindications to induction?
3. Dinoprostone is used for cervical ripening. What are the routes available for this medication? Identify specific instructions the nurse would provide to the client when administering each route.
4. Misoprostol is not formally approved for cervical ripening but remains one of the drugs used for it. However, it causes a higher incidence of uterine

tachysystole. What is this condition? This medication is given by tablet, but not by mouth. How is it administered when given for cervical ripening?

5. Oxytocin is used for the induction of labor near term. It has three pharmacologic effects. What are they?
6. Uterine rupture is a serious adverse effect of oxytocin administration. Which client populations are at specific risk for this while receiving oxytocin therapy? How does the nurse monitor the client to prevent this condition?
7. Identify the route and dosing used for oxytocin administration.

Tips for answering exam questions related to these medications (Rosenjack Burchum et al., 2016):

- Do not induce a client into labor if they have: umbilical cord prolapse, transverse fetal position, active genital herpes infection, previous caesarean delivery, history of myomectomy, or placenta previa.
- Cervical ripening MUST occur before labor can be safely induced. Drugs may be used to promote this such as dinoprostone and misoprostol
- The goal of oxytocin therapy is to gradually increase the dose until uterine contractions resembling those of spontaneous labor have been produced (contractions q 2-3 min lasting 45-60 seconds) (p.783).
- During oxytocin therapy mother's blood pressure, pulse rate and uterine contractility should be monitored. Fetus should be monitored for heart rate and rhythm.
- If maternal or fetal distress occurs during oxytocin administration stop the infusion- the contractions should diminish rapidly
- Complications that would warrant the termination of oxytocin therapy include: 1) elevation of resting uterine pressure above 15-20 mm Hg; 2) contractions that persist for more than 1 minute; 3) contractions that occur more often than 2-3 minutes and 4) pronounced alteration in fetal heart rate or rhythm (p.783).

DRUGS FOR POSTPARTUM HEMORRHAGE

1. What is the dosage of misoprostol when used to stop postpartum hemorrhage? By what route is it given (*differs from the previous route identified for cervical ripening*)? What are side effects of this medication?
2. Oxytocin is given IM or IV. Identify the dosing for both of these routes.
3. Carboprost tromethamine is the preferred agent for controlling postpartum hemorrhage (Rosenjack Burchum et al., 2016, p. 784). What is the route and dose of this medication? What are potential adverse effects of this medication?
4. Methylergonovine is only reserved for women who have not responded to oxytocin, misoprostol or carboprost tromethamine. This is due to its major adverse effect. What is it?

Tips for answering exam questions related to these medications (Rosenjack Burchum et al., 2016):

- Postpartum hemorrhage is defined as bleeding of any amount sufficient to cause hemodynamic instability (p.783)
- 80% of cases are caused by uterine atony. Other causes typically result from alterations, maternal coagulopathies or retention of placental tissue (p.783).
- Oxytocin is considered the first line agent for controlling postpartum hemorrhage
- Shivering and temperature elevation typically result from misoprostol administration (dosed rectally)
- Adverse effects are a primary area of focus for these drugs along with continuous assessment of hemodynamic stability in the mother

DRUGS FOR MENORRHAGIA

1. Tranexamic acid can decrease menstrual bleeding. What is its mechanism of action? Why would women be at risk of venous or arterial thrombosis when taking this medication?
2. How does NSAID therapy work to control menstrual bleeding?
3. What is the role of combination oral contraceptives in controlling menstrual bleeding?
4. What is the Levonorgestrel-Releasing Intrauterine System (Mirenva System)?

Tips for answering exam questions related to these medications (Rosenjack Burchum et al., 2016):

- Menorrhagia is defined as a period that lasts more than 7 days or if blood loss exceeds 80mLs
- The aim of all these medications is to decrease menstrual bleeding
- Iron deficiency anemia typically results from this condition. Signs of iron deficiency anemia include: decreased ferritin levels, decreased hemoglobin levels, decreased RBC size (decreased mean corpuscular volume).

Pediatric Considerations: Drugs and Breastfeeding

Drugs that are contraindicated during breastfeeding: methotrexate

Drugs of abuse that are contraindicated during breastfeeding: amphetamine, cocaine, heroin, marijuana, phencyclidine

Drugs with unknown effects on breastfeeding but may be of concern: metronidazole, amitriptyline, chlorpromazine, desipramine, diazepam, Haldol, imipramine. Trifluoperazine

Drugs that have been associated with significant effects on some breastfeeding infants and should be given to breastfeeding mothers with caution: aspirin, phenobarbital, ergotamine, lithium carbonate

Maternal medications usually compatible with breastfeeding: acetaminophen, ibuprofen, indomethacin, ketorolac tromethamine, mefenamic acid, naproxen, propoxyphene, acyclovir, amoxicillin, cefazolin, erythromycin, isoniazid, kanamycin, nitrofurantoin, streptomycin, sulfisoxazole, tetracycline, magnesium sulfate, phenytoin, atropine sulfate, propranolol, digoxin, hydralazine, methyldopa, nifedipine, quinidine, chlorothiazide, spironolactone, milk of magnesia, senna, estradiol, estrogen, insulin, levonogestrel, medroxyprogesterone, prednisone, progesterone, propylthiouracil, thyroxine, tolbutamide, codeine, meperidine, methadone, morphine, alcohol, caffeine, theophylline

PLEASE NOTE THAT THESE DRUGS WILL STILL INFLUENCE THE INFANT—OUTLINE ASSESSMENTS THE NURSE WOULD BE REQUIRED TO MAKE TO ENSURE THE INFANT IS SAFE DURING DRUG ADMINISTRATION

—American Academy of Pediatrics

PRACTICE QUESTIONS

Question 1
A client is receiving misoprostol for postpartum hemorrhage. The Health Care Provider has ordered 600 units rectally. What is a critical nursing intervention when administering this medication for postpartum hemorrhage?

1. The medication should be given orally instead of rectally
2. The medication is given after the delivery of the placenta
3. The medication is given after the delivery of the baby
4. The medication should be given intravenously instead of rectally

Question 2
A client is receiving terbutaline. Which of the following assessment findings related to the adverse effects of this medication would alert the nurse to contact the Health Care Provider immediately? **(Select all that apply)**

1. Coarse crackles auscultated throughout the client's lung fields
2. Blood pressure of 80/50 mmHg
3. Dizziness and flushing
4. Serum blood glucose level of 20 mmol/L
5. Elevated AST and ALT levels

Question 3
A 19-year-old client is receiving tranexamic acid for menorrhagia. Which of the following assessment findings would alert the nurse to a severe side effect associated with this medication?

1. Shortness of breath and expiratory wheezes on auscultation
2. Positive Homan's sign and increased serum D-dimer
3. Headache and back pain
4. Sinus and nasal congestion

Question 4
A 35-year-old client is experiencing a severe post-partum hemorrhage. Which of the following medications is the preferred treatment in this situation?

1. Oxytocin 40units in 1000mL IV fluid at 200mL/hr
2. Misoprostol 1000mcg rectally
3. Carboprost tromethamine 250mcg IM
4. Methylergonovine 0.2 mg IV prn

Question 5
A client is receiving oxytocin IV for induction of labor. Which of the following clinical findings would the nurse immediately stop the infusion for? **(Select all that apply)**

1. Resting uterine pressure above 15-20 mmHg
2. Maternal heart rate of 100 beats/ minute
3. Contractions that persist for more than 1 minute
4. Contractions that occur more often than every 2-3 minutes
5. Pronounced alteration in fetal heart rate or rhythm

Question 6
A client has been ordered to receive dinoprostone gel to encourage cervical ripening. The nurse administers 0.5mg/3mL dinoprostone gel intracervical. What instructions should the nurse provide to the client after administration of this medication?

1. To lie supine for 2 hours after pouch administration
2. To report any flushing or shortness of breath
3. To lie supine for at least 30 minutes after administration
4. To ensure that the mother counts fetal movements for 1 hour after medication administration

Answers: Question 1(2), Question 2(1,2,4), Question 3 (2), Question 4(3), Question 5(1,3,4,5), Question 6(3)

Study Strategy

This study guide differs from other resources because formal rationale is not provided for the answers. You need to determine the appropriate rationale for the correct answers by accessing the information in the question that may have inhibited your ability to answer the question correctly. It is helpful to ask the following questions:

- What is the question asking? What are key words in the question query?
- What information do I need to know to answer this question correctly?
- How did I select my answer?
- Why were the other answers incorrect?
- Was I missing a piece of content knowledge that inhibited how I answered the question? If so, what should I target in on and study?

Additional Strategies for Working with the Pharmacology Study Guide Modules

Content review is essential for being successful at answering NCLEX-RN® exam questions focusing on pharmacology. The following tips will help you to navigate the breath of this content and to organize your study notes. **Remember that you need to do the work of solid content review in order to be successful in understanding pharmacological concepts. Do not rely on practice questions to teach you what you need to know regarding medications for the NCLEX-RN®- practice questions are a tool for consolidating knowledge not a primary way to study.**

1. Complete the exercises in this study guide and make notes. This guide has been designed to direct you to important content for medication review. When creating the study guide I used an educator's lens to pull out the most important information in order ensure client safety with drug administration. For example, when review differing drugs I focused on critical information and essential education for each drug. The review questions are designed to bring this information forward.
2. Find ways to colour code or organize medications according to the bodily system or pathology they are used for. This will help you with recalling information. This guide uses a systems approach to help you organize the vast amount of pharmacological review in a way that will help you understand key concepts and pathologies.
3. Create case studies or unique ways to remember classes of medications. It is always wise to study pharmacology in the context of pathology. Use case studies specifically for content that is new to you or more difficult. Case studies should be memorable, contain client information that is easy to remember, focus on adverse effects of medications and key aspects of client education.

4. It is helpful to find patterns in names in drugs- such as suffixes that are common. Highlight the endings of common terms and find strategies to remember the main side effects of these classes of medications.
5. Client teaching is essential in medication administration. Ensure that you review your client education chapter in your Fundamentals of Nursing textbook (e.g. Potter and Perry). You need to remember that the use of basic teaching and learning principles paired with your knowledge of medications can help you to better exam questions.
6. When you use practice questions find consistent strategies for reviewing questions that you get incorrect. For example, the summary drug tables presented in each module of this guide provide a structure for organizing information. Create a blank table with the drug classes named for each system. Write information or content that is tested in each drug class as you move through your practice resources. Highlight the medication names you have seen in the practice questions on your summary table. Are there any patterns in the types of questions asked or the content tested? **Do be careful with this strategy- it is not a replacement for reviewing content.**

Conclusion

Strong pharmacological review will not only increase your chances of success on the NCLEX-RN® it will also strengthen your future nursing practice. The complexity of client care paired with the increase in co-morbidity and chronic disease management poses many challenges to pharmacological therapy. Nurses must be aware of potential drug-to-drug interactions, polypharmacy, and adverse events related to medications in order to keep their clients safe. I wish you all the best for your NCLEX-RN® exam and for your future nursing practice.

Best wishes,

Dr. Marnie Kramer-Kile

REFERENCES

Copstead, L.E & Banaski, J. (2013). *Pathophysiology* (5th ed). St. Louis: Elsevier.

Hogan, M. (2012). *Comprehensive review for NCLEX-RN®: Pearson reviews and rationales* (2nd ed.). New Jersey: Prentice Hall.

Rosenjack Burchum, J. & Rosenthal, L.D. (2016). *Lehne's pharmacology for nursing care* (9th edition). St. Louis: Elsevier.

Module 12

Pain Management and Anesthesia

TABLE OF CONTENTS

Introduction to the Transitioning to the NCLEX-RN® Pharmacology Guide: Pain Management and Anesthesia

The breadth and detail of the knowledge required of pharmacological concepts often overwhelms new graduates when they are beginning their exam preparation. The purpose of this pharmacology study guide is to help you work through the vast amount of pharmacological knowledge required for the NCLEX-RN® in a systematic and purposeful way. This guide organizes content using the current NCLEX-RN® Test Plan and provides specific strategies to address pharmacological areas of review which may challenge new graduates. **This is the twelfth of twelve modules.** This is a working guide, so while key information will be presented and organized for review, it is up to you to do the detailed work of content review by answering the questions and exercises in each section. You can expect to see drugs described by their generic names on the exam. Due to the differences in drug trade names between the United States of America, Canada and other nations you should study drugs according to their generic names and develop strategies for remembering them.

This module is part of a comprehensive pharmacology study guide focusing on specific areas which may challenge NCLEX-RN® candidates. This includes drug-to-drug interactions, specific adverse reactions due to drug therapy and the potential reactions associated with herbal therapy and conventional medications. The content will be focused on a systems approach and will direct you towards important information within each drug class.

Structure of the Module

This module begins with an overview of the drugs given for pain management and anesthesia. Additional areas for review that are specialized or affect multiple systems will also be highlighted:

1. Review questions and selected exercises will be constructed for each drug class to help pull out key concepts such as adverse events/side effects, specific client teaching and drug to drug interactions.
2. A summary chart of the drug classes in each system or theme will be provided for you to use alongside practice questions. As you move through practice questions, check off the specific medications you come across and if you require further review in each area. It is also helpful to make your own drug cards for specific medications. Keep the drug cards simple. Identify the drug class, the mechanism of action, two relevant (i.e., life threatening) or unique adverse effects that require monitoring and provide an outline for client teaching or specific nursing interventions for the medication.

Advice for Studying Pharmacological Content for the NCLEX-RN®

Always start with areas you are NOT familiar with. For example, if you spent the majority of your time as a final practicum student/or nurse on a cardiology unit do not start in the Vascular and Cardiac Medications Module. It is common for students/graduates to move to areas of comfort when they are studying because it decreases their anxiety. However, your efforts should be targeted on what you don't know. Each Module in this guide has a summary table of drugs for each system. Highlight the drug classes that you are not familiar with and make it your priority to work through them. Do not spend time making drug cards for medications you already know. For example, most students are confident with furosemide administration and can critically think through concepts associated with the drug. Therefore, time does not need to be spent studying this medication. Only make drug cards for medications that are new to you. The review questions in this guide will direct you towards more detailed information of the medications that you are familiar with and focus on potential areas where exam questions may be asked.

This guide is set up using a **systems approach** for the following reasons: 1) most pharmacology textbooks use this approach to structure content so it will be easier to find the information you need to answer the review questions; 2) using a systems approach allows you to find commonalties in the side effects of drugs influencing a specific system, so you will see patterns arising as you work through this guide; and 3) a systems approach allows for the creation of overall drug summary tables, which will be included in each module of the guide and will provide you with a general sense of the medications you need to cover.

The following resources will aid you in answering questions posed in this guide. This includes:

1. **A pharmacology textbook.** This resource will contain more detailed information pertaining to drug classes and outline general nursing considerations for therapy. I have referenced a pharmacology textbook throughout the writing of this guide.
2. **A drug guide**. These are the guides commonly used for your clinical practice. These resources contain alphabetized drug information. Most importantly, they outline specific pharmacokinetic and pharmacodynamics properties of drugs. You will find information related to drug excretion, protein binding, and therapeutic index in these guides.
3. **An online drug repository** for more detailed information that may not be found in the two resources above. Sometimes it is difficult to find therapeutic index and protein binding for a drug. I have found the following website helpful for this: http://www.drugbank.ca/drugs

Module 12: Pain Management and Anesthesia

This module addresses pain management and anesthesia. It is important to differentiate between analgesic and anesthesia because they are not synonymous terms. Analgesia refers to pain management and does not elicit unconsciousness, while anesthesia occurs in two major forms: 1) local anesthesia and 2) general anesthesia (inhaled and IV). Any type of anesthesia should always be accompanied by analgesia because pain management and client comfort is a primary concern. Analgesics also allow for lower dosing of anesthesia (p.258). Anesthesia in this module will be discussed primarily in the context of perioperative care. Table 12.1 outlines common medications in each of these contexts.

In order to fully understand the mechanism of action of opioids and anesthesia it is important to review key receptors that these drugs act on. In the case of opioid therapy the primary focus is on Mu and Kappa receptors.

When **Mu receptors** are activated they cause: analgesia, respiratory depression, sedation, euphoria, physical dependence and decreased GI motility (Rosenjack Burchum et al., 2016, p.261).

When **Kappa receptors** are activated they cause analgesia, sedation and decreased GI motility (p.261).

It is important to understand the agonist and antagonist relationships that certain drugs have with these receptors. This helps you to understand the complexity of drug-to-drug interactions and adverse effects related to different medication classes. Part 2 of this module explains the difference between pure opioid agonists, agonist-antagonist opioids and pure opioid antagonists.

When reviewing this content focus on the adverse events related to these medications. Think about these events in the context of your nursing assessments: How would a client present when experiencing these symptoms? What are expected nursing and medical interventions when these adverse events occur? What puts the client at an increased risk of experiencing adverse events?

The remainder of this module focuses on review questions related to anesthesia and pain management. Remember to make drug cards on at least one drug from each class. Start with drugs that you are unfamiliar with in the categories- for example, morphine is a common medication, start with other drugs in the same class that you have not had an opportunity to administer in clinical practice.

Table 12.1 Common Medications for Pain Management and Anesthesia

Medications for Anesthesia		
Topical Local Anesthetics Benzocaine Cocaine Dibucaine Dyclonine Lidocaine Pramoxine Tetracaine	**Injected Local Anesthetics** Bupivacaine Chloroprocaine Lidocaine Mepivacaine Prilocaine Procain Ropivacaine Tetracaine	**General Anesthetics** **Inhalation Anesthetics** Isoflurane Enflurane Desflurane Sevoflurane Nitrous oxide **Intravenous Anesthetics** Midazolam (benzodiazepine) Propofol Ketamine
Analgesics		
Pure Opioid Agonists Morphine Codeine Fentanyl Hydrocodone Hydromorphone Levophanol Meperidine Methadone Oxycodone Oxymorphone Remifentanil Sufentanil Tapentadol	**Agonist-Antagonist Opioids** Buprenorphine Butorphanol Nalbuphine Pentazocine **Drugs for Headache** Ergotamine Dihydroergotamine Almotriptan Eletriptan Frovatriptan Naratriptan Rizatriptan Sumatriptan Zolmitriptan	**NSAIDs** Aspirin Fenoprofen Ibuprofen Ketoprofen Naproxen Naproxen sodium Celecoxib Diflunisal Etodolac Meclofenamate sodium Mefenamic acid

PART ONE: ANESTHETICS

REVIEW QUESTIONS

TOPICAL LOCAL ANESTHETICS

Topical anesthetics are used administered topically or by injection (IV). All of these drugs have the potential for systemic toxicity. This may include cardiac toxicity (bradycardia, heart block, or cardiac arrest) or CNS toxicity (seizures, respiratory depression, coma)- the risk of toxicity increases with the amount absorbed (Rosenthal Burcham, 2016, p. 248). Most injections of local anesthetics are completed by an anesthesiologist (p.248).

1. How can the nurse prevent systemic toxicity of topical local anesthetics?
2. What is an adverse side effect of benzocaine in children 2 years or younger of age?

INJECTED LOCAL ANESTHETICS

1. What are noted side effects of bupivacaine? In which context is this drug commonly given?
2. What are signs of systemic reactions of local anesthetics given via injection?
3. Why must a history of allergy be associated with ester-type agents?

Tips for answering exam questions related to these medications (Rosenjack Burchum et al., 2016)

- Ester-type local anesthetics are contraindicated for clients with a history of serious allergies to these drugs
- Systemic toxicity is a primary concern- this is evidenced by cardiac suppression (bradycardia, heart blocks, cardiac arrest). If the client presents with any of these symptoms in the exam question it is a nursing priority to inform the Health Care Provider
- To avoid systemic toxicity the nurse applies a minimal amount (for effect) of a topical local anesthetic and never applies the medication over injured skin.
- Topical benzocaine can cause methemoglobinemia that can result in death. Look up symptoms of this condition- it is also a rare side effect of nitroglycerin administration as well.
- Injected local anesthetics are given for surgical, dental and obstetric procedures and given my Health Care Providers with special training
- Bupivacaine is commonly given in epidural therapy during labour. It can cause bradycardia and CNS depression in the newborn

- Pain responses are decreased so clients may not recognize complications occurring in their body- special assessment needs to be completed to ensure client safety.

GENERAL ANESTHETICS (INHALED AND INJECTED)

1. Complete the following table outlining adverse effects of inhaled anesthetics as a group:

Adverse Effect	Description of Signs and Symptoms
Respiratory Depression	
Cardiac Depression	
Sensitization of heart to catecholamines	
Malignant Hyperthermia	
Aspiration of Gastric Contents	
Hepatotoxicity	
Toxicity to Operating Room Personnel	

2. Why are the following drugs given as adjuncts to inhalation anesthesia?
   a. Benzodiazepines (midazolam)
   b. Opioids (morphine and fentanyl)
   c. $Alpha_2$-Adrenergic Agonists (clonidine, dexmedetomidine)
   d. Anticholinergic drugs (atropine)
   e. Neuromuscular blocking agents (succinylcholine, pancuronium)
3. Why are the following postanesthetic medications given?
   a. Analgesics (morphine)
   b. Antiemetics (promethazine and droperidol)
   c. Muscarinic agonists (bethanechol)

4. Diazepam, lorazepam and midazolam are administered IV for induction of anesthesia. What are adverse effects related to each of these medications?
5. Propofol is a widely used IV anesthetic. What are the two most serious adverse effects of this medication? Why is this drug linked to higher rates of infection?
6. Ketamine produces dissociative anesthesia. What does this mean? What are adverse psychologic reactions associated with this drug?

Tips for answering exam questions related to these medications (Rosenjack Burchum et al., 2016, p.258)

- Inhalation anesthetics are eliminated almost entirely in expired air
- Client often require mechanical ventilation when receiving this drug therapy
- Co-administration of succinylcholine with general anesthetics increases the risk of malignant hyperthermia in those clients with a genetic risk for this condition
- Nitrous oxide is not a potent anesthetic and is often co-administered with other medications
- Clients recovering from ketamine may have adverse psychologic reactions
- Medications such as benzodiazepines, opioids and anticholinergic medications are given 30-60 minutes prior to general anesthesia.

PART TWO: PAIN MANAGEMENT

Nociception: Physiologic mechanisms involved in the pain phenomenon which are divided into four stages:

Transduction, 2) Transmission, 3) Perception and 4) Modulation

Table 12.2 Basic Physiology of Pain

Transduction

The process of converting painful stimuli to neuronal action potentials at the sensory receptor

(Stimulation can occur from direct damage to nerve endings or from the release of chemical mediators such as K+, H+, lactate, histamine, prostaglandins, serotonin, and bradykinins at the site of injury)

Nociceptors stimulated	Noxious stimuli transduced into neuronal action potentials	Action potentials travel through spinal tract and then into the brain

Transmission

The movement of action potentials along neurons that make their way from the peripheral receptor to the spinal cord and then centrally to the brain

Stimulation of CNS through sensory fibers

A-Delta Fibers	C-Fibers
Fast transmission mylenated nerves	Slow transmission mylenated nerves
Sharp, stinging, cutting, pinching pain	Dull, burning, aching pain
Source: Thermal, mechanical stimuli	Source: Polymodal stimuli (mechanical, thermal, chemical)
	Projects to areas of brain that produce displeasure, anxiety

These A-Delta and C-Fibers enter the dorsal horn of the spinal cord, synapsing on interneurons within the spinal cord, crossing to the opposite side and traveling to the brain via the anterolateral tract. These pain signals are carried to the brain through the use of various neurotransmitters and neuropeptides. An example of this is substance P. The neurotransmitters bind to the next neurons in the pathway and thereby initiate action potentials, interruption of these synaptic processes can inhibit pain transmission.

Note: Anterolateral tract (also known as the spinothalmic tract) has two divisions: 1) neospinothalamic tract and the paleospinothalamic tract. **Neospinothalamic** division has fewer synapse in the cord and projects first to the thalamus, A-delta fibers use this tract as it reaches the brain quickly to provide the brain about pain location, but there is little emotional connection.
Paleospinothalmic tract has a greater number of synapses and reaches the brain more slowly. C-fibers travel mainly in this tract and as a result stirs aversive emotional responses (Copstead et al., 2010, p.1108). This pain is poorly localized, longer lasting and more distressing.

Perception
Occurs when the brain receives pain signals and interprets them as painful

Perception includes: awareness, interpretation of meaning and sensation. Pain perception is not localized to a particular brain area. Pain perception is described in terms of pain threshold and pain tolerance.

Pain threshold: level of painful stimulation required to be perceived and is similar from one individual to another

Pain tolerance: the degree of pain that one is willing to bear before seeking relief.

Pain expression: is the way in which the pain experiences are communicated to others (Copstead et al., 2010, p.1109).

Modulation
The complex mechanism whereby synaptic transmission of pain signals is altered

Occurs at multiple sites among pain pathway.

Modulation of pain at the level of the spinal cord:
Main theory regarding ascending pathways is the Gate Control Theory of Pain (Melzack & Wall, 1965): Rubbing, pressing, or shaking painful area may reduce the intensity of pain at the level of the spinal cord.
Theories regarding descending pathways from brain to dorsal horn surround the use of opioid analgesics to prevent the signal of pain going back to the site of injury.

Modulation of pain at the level of the brain: Specific opioid receptors have been discovered in the brain, as well as endorphins. Specific opioid receptors called Mu and Kappa receptors have analgesic activities when they are activated by opioid analgesics. These are found in high concentration within the brain, where they are thought to modulate pain perception. Kappa receptors also have analgesic effects and are found in high concentrations within the spinal cord, where they help with pain modulation within descending CNS pathways.

It is helpful to use the following framework when thinking about pain management and the selection of appropriate medications.

World Health Organization Analgesic Ladder

Step 1-Mild pain (e.g.: NSAIDS or acetaminophen)

Step 2-Moderate pain-add weaker opioids-limited by the ceiling effects

Step 3-Severe pain-stronger opioids (e.g. morphine)

Step 4-Intractable pain-nerve blocks or even anesthetics

Consequences of unmanaged pain can result in (Lewis et al., 2014):

- Increased oxygen demand
- Respiratory dysfunction
- Decreased GI motility
- Confusion
- Depressed immune system
- Anxiety, depression

REVIEW QUESTIONS

OPIOID MEDICATIONS

PURE OPIOID AGONISTS

These medications activate mu and kappa receptors. They are considered agonists. Morphine is a prototype drug for a strong agonist, while codeine is considered a moderate to strong agonist (p.251).

1. Outline the most common adverse effects associated with opioid medications:

Adverse Effect	Assessment Required and Treatment
Respiratory Depression	
Constipation	
Orthostatic hypotension	
Urinary Retention	

Cough suppression	
Biliary Colic	
Emesis	
Elevation of ICP	
Euphoria/Dysphoria	
Sedation	
Miosis	

Tips for answering exam questions related to these medications (Rosenjack Burchum et al., 2016, pp.281-283)

- Oral morphine doses are higher than parental doses because of the first pass effect of the liver
- Infants require smaller dosing of opioids because the blood-brain barrier is poorly developed
- With prolonged opioid use tolerance will develop for analgesia, euphoria, sedation, and respiratory depression- NOT constipation or miosis
- Withdrawal syndrome associated with morphine is unpleasant but not dangerous- as with other CNS depressants
- Opioid overdose is characterized by: coma, respiratory depression and pinpoint pupils
- Meperidine use should not exceed past 48hrs- a toxic metabolite builds up (normeperidine)
- Combination of codeine with a nonopioid analgesic produces greater pain relief than when administered alone.
- Opioids are contraindicated or all **premature infants (during and after delivery)**
- Morphine is contraindicated following biliary tract surgery
- Meperidine is contraindicated for clients taking MAOIs

AGONIST-ANTAGONIST OPIOIDS

There are four drugs in this class available (Table 12.1) when given alone they produce analgesia, when given with a pure opioid agonist they counteract the effects of the agonist drug (p.261). For example, if a client is receiving pentazocine if they are also given morphine (opioid agonist) the pentazocine will diminish the effects of the morphine.

1. Most agonist-antagonist opioids have a ceiling effect with respiratory depression. What does this mean for the client?
2. Why is the risk of abuse low in this class of medications?
3. What assessment findings can the nurse expect if a agonist-antagonist opioid is administered with a pure opioid agonist?

Tips for answering exam questions related to these medications (Rosenjack Burchum et al., 2016, p.285)

- Do not give this class of medications to clients with acute myocardial infarction because they cause increased cardiac workload
- These medication can cause abstinence syndrome in clients taking other opioids because of their antagonist properties
- Maximal pain relief is lower in this class of drugs than with pure opioid agonists
- These medications have a lower potential for abuse

PURE OPIOID ANTAGONISTS

This drug class includes **naloxone**- this drug is an antagonist for mu and kappa receptors and will reverse the effects of all pure opioid medications. Naloxone must be used with caution, reversal of opioids can cause rebound pain and precipitate withdrawal in clients addicted to opiates.

NSAIDs

Non-steroidal anti-inflammatory drugs (NSAIDs) are given for pain management and as adjunctive therapy to opioids. NSAIDs work on the cyclo-oxygenase 1 and 2 enzymes. See Figure 12.1 below.

Non-Steroidal Anti-Inflammatory Drugs (NSAIDS)

1st Generation NSAIDS (inhibit COX1 and COX2)

2Nd Generation NSAIDS (inhibit COX2)

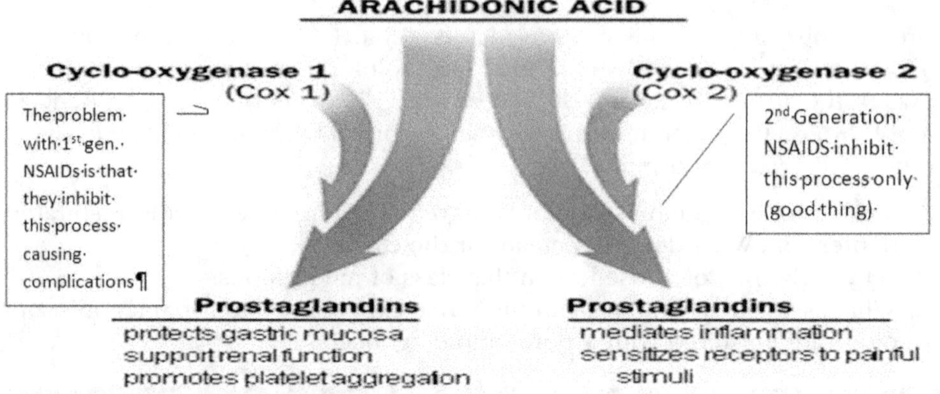
ARACHIDONIC ACID
Cyclo-oxygenase 1
(Cox 1)
Cyclo-oxygenase 2
(Cox 2)
The problem with 1st gen. NSAIDs is that they inhibit this process causing complications
2nd Generation NSAIDS inhibit this process only (good thing)
Prostaglandins
protects gastric mucosa
support renal function
promotes platelet aggregation
Prostaglandins
mediates inflammation
sensitizes receptors to painful stimuli

Figure 12.1 NSAID therapy and cyclo-oxygenase enzyme inhibition

1. What is the difference between first and second generation NSAID therapy?
2. What are common side effects associated with first generation NSAIDs?
3. How is an aspirin overdose treated?
4. What are signs of salicylism?
5. What is Reye's syndrome and how it is associated with aspirin therapy? Who is at risk of developing this condition?
6. How does long term aspirin use affect the kidneys?
7. Why is Celecoxib contraindicated for clients with a sulfa allergy?
8. Which client populations should NSAIDs be used with caution in?
9. Outline GI reactions associated with NSAID therapy.
10. What is the treatment for an acetaminophen overdose?

Tips for answering exam questions related to these medications (Rosenjack Burchum et al., 2016, p.866-868)

- Aspirin induced gastric ulcers can be reduced by testing and eliminating H.pylori before starting therapy and by giving a proton pump inhibitor or H2 receptor antagonist.
- Ibuprofen, naproxen and other nonaspirin NSAIDs can antagonize the anti-platelet actions of aspirin; clients should take aspirin 2 hours before other NSAIDs
- Discard aspirin preparations that smell like vinegar (p.866).
- High dose aspirin should be discontinued 7-10 days before elective surgery. It does not need to be stopped for dental surgery, dermatologic or cataract surgeries.

- Low dose aspirin should be continued in 1) clients undergoing coronary artery bypass surgery, clients considered high risk of a cardiovascular event who require noncardiac surgery or percutaneous coronary intervention.
- Keep NSAID doses low in clients with renal insufficiency
- Nonaspirin NSAIDs (not Aspirin itself) increase the risk of MI and stroke.
- NSAIDs (including acetaminophen) may blunt the immune response to vaccines- advise parents to avoid routine use of NSAIDs to prevent vaccination-associated fever and pain
- Advise patients who are undernourished (e.g. owing to fasting or illness) to consume no more than 3000mg of acetaminophen a day (p.868).

DRUGS FOR HEADACHE

Drug therapy for headache is focused on either 1) aborting an existing attack or 2) preventing a future attack.

1. Sumatriptan is a serotonin receptor agonist (triptan) and a first line agent for aborting a migraine headache. It is given sc or intranasally. What are adverse effects related to this medication? Which client populations should these medications NOT be given to?
2. Aspirin when combined with which other drug has the same therapeutic effects as sumatriptan?
3. Ergotamine is a second-line agent for stopping an ongoing migraine attack in clients who have not responded to sumatriptan. It potentially causes a toxicity known as ergotism in clients who overdose on this medication. What are the signs of this condition?
4. Which client populations is ergotamine administration contraindicated for?
5. **Preventative therapy** for migraines includes: beta blockers, antiepileptic drugs (divalproex, topiramate), tricyclic antidepressants, estrogens and triptans. Outline how each of these drug classes work for the treatment of migraines.

Tips for answering exam questions related to these medications (Rosenjack Burchum et al., 2016)

- Meperidine and butorphanol nasal spray are preferred opioid analgesics given for migraine headaches. Butorphanol is the preferred drug because it does not precipitate opioid side effects on mu and kappa receptors to the same extent that meperidine does.
- Erotamine is well tolerated at usual therapeutic doses, it can stimulate the CTZ causing nausea and vomiting- typically metoclopramide is given concurrently with this drug
- Advise client to rest in a quiet dark room for 2-3 hours after drug administration and apply an ice pack to the neck and scalp.
- Educate clients to eliminate stress factors.

PRACTICE QUESTIONS

Question 1
Which of the following is a consequence of unmanaged pain?

1. Decreased oxygen demand.
2. Decreased gastrointestinal activity.
3. Hyperactivity.
4. Increased immune response.

Question 2
Which of the following statements is true regarding chronic regular dosing of narcotic analgesics?

1. Constipation disappears after about two weeks of use.
2. Their major action is peripheral.
3. Sedation and drowsiness are side effects which increase with long-term continuous use.
4. Co-administration with non-narcotic analgesics may provide additive analgesic effects without increasing narcotic dose.

Question 3
When administering morphine sulphate which of the following assessment findings would indicate a *serious* side effect of this medication?

1. Respiratory Rate of 16 breaths per minute
2. Blood pressure of 102/80 mmHg
3. Urine output less than 30cc per hour
4. Itching on the patient's face and nose

Question 4
Morphine sulphate 5mg IV q2-4h prn has been ordered for Denise by the physician. Which opioid receptors in the body does morphine act on in order to produce its analgesic effects?

1. Mu and Delta receptors
2. Kappa and Delta receptors
3. Mu and Kappa receptors
4. Alpha and Mu receptors

Question 5
A client has a known family history of malignant hyperthermia with the administration of general anesthetic. Which of the following medications puts the client at an increased risk of developing this condition when administered with general anesthesia?

1. Pancuronium
2. Morphine
3. Warfarin
4. Succinylcholine

Question 6
A client with a history of migraine headaches is taking Erotamine to abort acute headaches when they occur. Which drug is recommended as an adjunct to treat the side effects of Erotamine?

1. Metoclopramide
2. Dimenhydrinate
3. Ondanestron
4. Ibuprofen

Answers: Question 1(2), Question 2(4), Question 3 (3), Question 4(3), Question 5(4), Question 6(1)

Study Strategy

This study guide differs from other resources because formal rationale is not provided for the answers. You need to determine the appropriate rationale for the correct answers by accessing the information in the question that may have inhibited your ability to answer the question correctly. It is helpful to ask the following questions:

- What is the question asking? What are key words in the question query?
- What information do I need to know to answer this question correctly?
- How did I select my answer?
- Why were the other answers incorrect?
- Was I missing a piece of content knowledge that inhibited how I answered the question? If so, what should I target in on and study?

Additional Strategies for Working with the Pharmacology Study Guide Modules

Content review is essential for being successful at answering NCLEX-RN® exam questions focusing on pharmacology. The following tips will help you to navigate the breath of this content and to organize your study notes. **Remember that you need to do the work of solid content review in order to be successful in understanding pharmacological concepts. Do not rely on practice questions to teach you what you need to know regarding medications for the NCLEX-RN®- practice questions are a tool for consolidating knowledge not a primary way to study.**

1. Complete the exercises in this study guide and make notes. This guide has been designed to direct you to important content for medication review. When creating the study guide I used an educator's lens to pull out the most important information in order ensure client safety with drug administration. For example, when review differing drugs I focused on critical information and essential education for each drug. The review questions are designed to bring this information forward.
2. Find ways to colour code or organize medications according to the bodily system or pathology they are used for. This will help you with recalling information. This guide uses a systems approach to help you organize the vast amount of pharmacological review in a way that will help you understand key concepts and pathologies.
3. Create case studies or unique ways to remember classes of medications. It is always wise to study pharmacology in the context of pathology. Use case studies specifically for content that is new to you or more difficult. Case studies should be memorable, contain client information that is easy to remember, focus on adverse effects of medications and key aspects of client education.

4. It is helpful to find patterns in names in drugs- such as suffixes that are common. Highlight the endings of common terms and find strategies to remember the main side effects of these classes of medications.
5. Client teaching is essential in medication administration. Ensure that you review your client education chapter in your Fundamentals of Nursing textbook (e.g. Potter and Perry). You need to remember that the use of basic teaching and learning principles paired with your knowledge of medications can help you to better exam questions.
6. When you use practice questions find consistent strategies for reviewing questions that you get incorrect. For example, the summary drug tables presented in each module of this guide provide a structure for organizing information. Create a blank table with the drug classes named for each system. Write information or content that is tested in each drug class as you move through your practice resources. Highlight the medication names you have seen in the practice questions on your summary table. Are there any patterns in the types of questions asked or the content tested? **Do be careful with this strategy- it is not a replacement for reviewing content.**

Conclusion

Strong pharmacological review will not only increase your chances of success on the NCLEX-RN® it will also strengthen your future nursing practice. The complexity of client care paired with the increase in co-morbidity and chronic disease management poses many challenges to pharmacological therapy. Nurses must be aware of potential drug-to-drug interactions, polypharmacy, and adverse events related to medications in order to keep their clients safe. I wish you all the best for your NCLEX-RN® exam and for your future nursing practice.

Best wishes,

Dr. Marnie Kramer-Kile

REFERENCES

Adams, M.P., Holland, L.N., Bostwick, P.M. & King (2010). *Pharmacology for nurses: A pathophysiologic approach* (Canadian ed). Toronto, ON: Pearson.

Copstead, L.C. & Banasik, J. L. (2010). *Pathophysiology* (4th ed.). St. Louis: Elsevier Canada.

Copstead, L.E & Banaski, J. (2013). *Pathophysiology* (5th ed). St. Louis: Elsevier.

Day, R., Paul, P., Williams, B., Smeltzer, S., & Bare, B. (2007). *Brunner & Suddarth's textbook of medical-surgical Nursing*. Philadelphia: Lippincott Williams & Wilkins.

Jovey, R.D et al. (2002). *Managing pain: The Canadian healthcare professional's reference*. The Canadian Pain Society.

Rosenjack Burchum, J. & Rosenthal, L.D. (2016). *Lehne's pharmacology for nursing care* (9th edition). St. Louis: Elsevier.

www.ingramcontent.com/pod-product-compliance
Lightning Source LLC
Chambersburg PA
CBHW070223190526
45169CB00001B/55